Epidemiology as a Fundamental Science

EPIDEMI

This is the report of a conference sponsored
by the Health Resources Administration of
the U.S. Department of Health, Education and
Welfare that was organized by the International
Epidemiological Association and held
on March 2–4, 1975.

OLOGY

AS A FUNDAMENTAL SCIENCE

Its Uses in Health Services Planning, Administration, and Evaluation

Edited by

Kerr L. White, M.D.
Professor of Health Care Organization
The Johns Hopkins University
School of Hygiene and Public Health

Maureen M. Henderson, M.D.
Assistant Vice-President for Health Affairs
Health Services Center
University of Washington

With a Foreword by
Kenneth M. Endicott, M.D.

New York

Oxford University Press

1976

This volume and the conference on which it is based were made
possible by the support of the Health Resources Administration of
the United States Department of Health, Education and Welfare under
Contract No. HRA 230-75-0091.

Planning Committee

Lynne S. Apostolides
(Conference Coordinator and
    Technical Editor)
Consultant, International Epide-
    miological Association

John C. Greene
Chief Dental Officer
Public Health Service
and
Special Assistant for Dental Affairs
Office of the Assistant Secretary
    for Health
Department of Health, Education
    and Welfare

Theodore C. Haaser
Vice-President
Rosslyn Foundation
Silver Spring, Maryland

Maureen M. Henderson
Assistant Vice-President for Health
    Affairs
Health Services Center
University of Washington
Seattle, Washington

William A. Lybrand
Associate Administrator for Scien-
    tific Affairs
Office of Scientific Affairs
Health Resources Administration
Department of Health, Education
    and Welfare

Louis M. F. Massé
Professor
Ecole Nationale de la Santé
    Publique
Rennes, France

Thomas McCarthy
Acting Deputy Administrator for
 Scientific Affairs
Office of Scientific Affairs
Health Resources Administration
Department of Health, Education
 and Welfare

Edward B. Perrin
Professor of Biostatistics
University of Washington
Seattle, Washington

Gerald Rosenthal
Director
National Center for Health Services
 Research
Health Resources Administration
Department of Health, Education
 and Welfare

James Shanks
President
Rosslyn Foundation
Silver Spring, Maryland

W. Estlin Waters
Professor and Head
Department of Community
 Medicine
University of Southampton Medi-
 cal School
Southampton, England

Kerr L. White
(Chairman)
Professor of Health Care Organi-
 zation
The Johns Hopkins University
 School of Hygiene and Public
 Health
Baltimore, Maryland

Virginia Williams
Office of Scientific Affairs
Health Resources Administration
Department of Health, Education
 and Welfare

Daniel I. Zwick
Associate Administrator for Plan-
 ning, Evaluation and Legislation
Office of Planning, Evaluation and
 Legislation
Health Resources Administration
Department of Health, Education
 and Welfare

Foreword

The Health Resources Administration of the United States Department of Health, Education and Welfare has been given substantial new responsibilities for assisting the states and their localities in planning health services and in allocating health care resources. Implementation of these activities necessarily will involve utilization of data and information specifically relevant to planning purposes. Prior to embarking upon major new data and information collection efforts, it is critical that available relevant data and information be assembled and used to best advantage. This effort will need to be carefully synchronized with the data and information activities of Professional Standards Review Organizations, Utilization Review Committees, and Medicare-Medicaid reporting systems. All of the above must be done in the context of recent federal legislation which calls for the establishment of the Cooperative Federal-State-Local Health Statistics System.

Clearly, proper execution of this task will require broad understanding of the concepts generated by epidemiologists and health statisticians, and by related disciplines, as well as widespread use of their methods.

Health decision-making issues can be better illuminated, and choices more fully informed, through clear expression of practical measurements of needs, resources, use, outcomes, and costs—and we should make the effort to do so. No longer can the United States, with an annual expenditure of upwards of one hundred and fifteen billion dollars on health care, afford the luxury of postponing the full development and the application of knowledge and skills which are directly relevant to understanding and coping with a critical national phenomenon.

It was toward this end that the Health Resources Administration sponsored the conference on which this volume is based. I hope that it will be widely read and that it will both promote understanding and stimulate appropriate action.

Kenneth M. Endicott, M.D.
Administrator
Health Resources Administration

June 1, 1976

Preface

This compendium of papers seeks to illustrate some of the potential contributions of quantitative approaches to the problems of allocating finite resources with the object of improving the public's health. These quantitative approaches are largely embodied in the concepts, principles, and methods embraced by the disciplines of epidemiology and health statistics, and their intellectual cousins, demography and sociology. The public policy problems and issues surrounding the allocation of limited health care resources have been accentuated in the United States by widespread concern about rapidly escalating costs, uneven access to services, duplication of sophisticated technical resources, and by doubts about the quality and value of many preventive, diagnostic, and therapeutic services. The emphasis on therapeutic and technical rather than on preventive and educational approaches is also being widely questioned. Such concerns have found public expression in recent federal legislation dealing with health planning, health statistics, health services research, and peer review of the quality of care; inevitably, there will be analogous legislation dealing with health manpower, especially with the balanced provision not only of specialized but also of primary or general medical care, and eventually with national health insurance.

It was the purpose of the editors and the Planning Committee to draw attention to both the opportunities of and the constraints on the fulfilment of congressional intent at the present juncture. The opportunities for introducing quantitative methods in the planning, administration, and evaluation of health services are reflected in the frequent legislative references to populations, communities, and information systems, all of which involve the use of concepts and methods fundamental to the disciplines of epidemiology and health statistics. It is simply not going to be feasible to implement the intent of the legislation without the use of ideas and measurements derived from epidemiological and statistical approaches and practices. The constraints, on the other hand, that may frustrate the national legislative intent, are the results of widespread ignorance or lack of appreciation, especially among the health care establishment and among policy-makers concerned with health matters, of the underlying concepts and quantitative relationships that could provide facts and estimates. It is these which could improve the climate of decision making with respect to resource allocation for health and health services. In addition, there is a serious scarcity of epidemiologists and health statisticians capable of tackling the problems reflected in the current legislation and of furthering the attainment of the objectives specified or implied. The scarcity is present at both practice and training levels and will be aggravated unless current trends of recruitment are reversed.

The contributions of this compendium are designed to illustrate the concepts of epidemiology as a fundamental science in health services planning, administration, and evaluation, and to document both the present state of affairs and the projected needs for epidemiologists and health statisticians. To accomplish its purpose, the planners of this volume were able to take advantage of the presence in the United States of the Council of the International Epidemiological Association, a scientific organization of some six hundred members in over sixty countries. The Council Members bring a wealth of national and international experiences from both governmental and academic settings to bear on the problems under discussion, and can illustrate their points with practical applications from diverse settings. These international perspectives and traditions, while not always transferable to the American setting, are nonetheless relevant to this country, since they demonstrate both the opportunities and the constraints that have been faced, and that are continually being faced elsewhere, in the struggle to improve the health and limit the disability and dependence of individuals and populations.

The introductory papers by Evans and McKeown provide the overall theme for this volume—a theme based on scientific evidence and pragmatic concern for relating benefits experienced to efforts expended, or of relating value received to money spent in the contexts of political and biological realities. Two major contributions discuss the theoretical and practical applications of epidemiology in allocating health resources in Canada and the United Kingdom. These are followed by discussions of opportunities, needs, and resources for the application of epidemiology and health statistics in the United States. The practical problems faced in a variety of settings are presented in the balance of the papers, with comments on each group by a discussant from the United States.

Detailed discussions of the papers, and of the problems and issues that emerge from them, have been summarized, and a final statement reflecting the sense of the participants concludes the volume. In no sense does this reflect the "official" position of any formal organization or body, but it does express the view of an experienced group of people from governmental, organizational, foundation, and academic settings, who reviewed the evidence, debated the problems and issues, and reached a general conclusion. As such, it is hoped that this volume will contribute not only to the debate, but also to constructive action that will improve the planning, administration, and evaluation of health services.

Kerr L. White, M.D.
Maureen M. Henderson, M.D.

Baltimore, Maryland
June 1, 1976

Contents

I

INTRODUCTION

1
JOHN R. EVANS, M.D.

PLANNING AND EVOLUTION IN CANADIAN HEALTH POLICY AND PROGRAMS

Basic problems in the health field are similar in Canada and the United States, but since World War II quite different health policies have evolved in the two countries. The United States strategy was much bolder in that it attempted to eliminate disease through research. Primary emphasis in government spending was given to the support of medical sciences. In Canada, on the other hand, relatively less support was given to scientific research and major emphasis was put on the elimination of financial barriers to health services and improvement of the resources for the delivery of health care. A second difference was the broad Canadian acceptance at an early stage of major direct governmental participation in health services while the United States continued to rely primarily on private initiatives and institutions. This latter difference in approach may reflect in part a fundamental distinction in attitude toward government in the two countries. The third major difference surrounds the opportunity for public involvement. Under Canada's constitution, health is primarily a provincial responsibility and, as a result, programs evolved in small, more manageable jurisdictions close to those served. The development of programs in different provinces varied in timing in relation to local needs and attitudes. The Federal Government has, of necessity, played mainly a coordinating role, and, through the mechanism of financial incentives and assistance, has minimized disparities in resources among the provinces.

The chronology of development of health policy in Canada reflects a slow, staged sequence of steps taken over more than two decades. In 1945 a comprehensive plan for publicly supported health services was developed by the Federal Government and supported by the Canadian Medical Association. Two features of this plan were health insurance and health centers. The first intervention by the Federal Government in the health scene was the establishment of the National Health Grants in 1948. One of the most important aspects of this program was the support of hospital construction in preparation for national hospital insurance. During the 1950's several provinces introduced hospital insurance and in 1958 the national plan was established. Following on the report of the Royal Commission on Health Services a federal health resources fund was established in 1965 to assist the provinces in upgrading and expanding facilities for education of the health professions and for medical research. This plan recognized the need to supply more doctors, dentists, and other health workers in anticipation of the introduction of medical care insurance, which Saskatchewan was the first province to introduce in 1962. Medical care insurance was enacted by the Federal Government in 1969 and fully adopted by all provinces by 1970. Since 1970 Canadians have had universal, publicly administered, prepaid health insurance. All necessary medical and hospital services, except dental services and prescription drugs, are covered and there are no limits on benefits provided. The health plans are financed primarily from tax revenues, although some provinces impose premiums related to the level of taxable income. The introduction of national health insurance has not been associated with any change in the ownership of hospitals or in the private practice of medicine. Nine out of ten hospitals are still owned and operated by private boards and there is no distinction between private and public hospital beds other than nonmedical amenities for which supplementary insurance can be obtained. Similarly, there is no distinction between private medical practice and practice under the publicly sponsored health insurance plan. Doctors are not civil servants, and most practitioners are paid for both hospital and office work on a fee-for-service basis in accordance with a fee schedule negotiated between the government and each provincial medical association.

Two questions are frequently asked about the Canadian system. First, did medicare and hospital insurance lead to a great increase in utilization of services? The answer is "no." There was a small increase immediately after the introduction of each plan but no increase was sustained, that is, there was no change in the pattern of increasing utilization of services evident before the publicly sponsored insurance plans were introduced. It should be pointed out, however, that programs to increase the number of hospital beds through construction grants and to increase the supply of health personnel were introduced in preparation for hospital and medical care insurance and these programs resulted in significant increases in operating costs. The second question is whether medicare actually did increase the accessibility of health services. Studies carried out in Quebec and in Saskatchewan did show a shift in the population served, with increased use of the services by those in lower income categories. In certain provinces, New Brunswick and Newfoundland for example, an increase in the number of physicians entering practice in the province appeared to be associated with the introduction of health insurance. This movement may be explained either by the increase in supply of physicians or by the fact that practice in economically marginal areas now became financially viable because all the patients were covered by health insurance.

Has medical care insurance solved the major problems of the Canadian health care system? It has certainly overcome financial barriers which limited access to medical care. It has not, however, solved the problems of geographic accessibility, the imbalance between active treatment hospital beds and other types of health facilities for chronic, convalescent, and ambulatory care, containment of costs, control of quality, or overemphasis on the management of disease rather than the promotion of health. Although national health insurance has not solved any of these problems, it has resulted in broad public recognition of these problems and transferred responsibility for leadership in the amelioration of the problems from the individual to government. That is, it has forced public acceptance of responsibility for health services.

What instruments were used to direct the pattern of development of health services in Canada? As I noted earlier, a reasonably comprehensive plan was developed shortly after World War II and early in the 1960's the Royal Commission on Health Services presented a comprehensive review of needs and recommended a broad range of programs to achieve a health plan for the nation. The instruments selected to implement these plans were not on the same broad comprehensive scale. The principal instrument of development was a financing mechanism established to retain expensive health facilities which could no longer be made available or kept up to date through local support and philanthropy. This was particularly true of active treatment hospital services. The mechanism also abolished financial barriers to health care, that is, made services accessible without regard to the income of the recipient. The tools of hospital construction grants and hospital and medical care insurance were too blunt to develop a balanced program of health services. They inevitably led to imbalance through overgrowth of some services and facilities and neglect of others. The second instrument in the health plan was development of educational resources to train more health personnel and promote health research. One major limitation in accessibility of health services was deemed to be an inadequate supply of health manpower. Following on the Royal Commission on Health Services a health resources development program was established to increase the educational capacity of our health training programs in universities and colleges. However, as other jurisdictions have learned, the increase in supply of health personnel did not solve the inequities of geographic distribution of health personnel, the imbalance between medical specialists and generalists, and the problems of interrelationships of medical and dental personnel with members of the allied health professions.

It has now been recognized that the manipulation of educational programs, that is, the supply side of the health manpower equation, is not necessarily sufficient in itself to achieve specific manpower benefits for the system of health services. Controls at the utilization level may be necessary to achieve intended health benefits without exorbitant cost. In some regions of Canada a good deal of success has resulted from the use of service incentives in underserviced areas. Return of service bursaries or indenture has also been used. But incentives and indenture only deal with areas of shortage of supply and it is now apparent that we also need a mechanism to handle areas in which there is a surplus or oversupply of physicians. Although a surplus may be attractive at first sight, it is now clear that an excess of doctors, particularly of those whose practice is hospital-bed based and heavily dependent on procedures, may significantly increase health costs without improving measures of health or health care. The prospect of a significant oversupply of doctors has precipitated changes in national immigration regulations to restrict inflow except where there is established need, and in some areas has led to consideration of the introduction of some type of "establishment" or upper limits on the number of physicians by type of practice in a geographic region. The concept of a regional "establishment" of physicians could help to produce an optimal distribution of general practitioners and specialists; it could be used to link changes in medical manpower to the evolution of patterns of practice and the involvement of other types of health personnel; and it could be a major factor in achieving control of costs. The third and most recently introduced instrument in the health plan is planning and organization of health services at the regional or district level. At the outset there was no framework within which institutions, agencies, and health personnel could coordinate their efforts to deliver health services. Organization per se had been used as an instrument exclusively at the provincial government level, a level too gross to achieve the balancing and coordination of health services in relation to local and regional needs. The scene is now changing with new efforts to organize regional and local health services on a comprehensive basis. The desirability of regional or district control of the planning and operation of health services has been accepted in principle in all provinces of Canada, but intermediate structures for administering health services at the regional level have only been developed in Quebec.

Appointed regional and district health councils have been hampered in their impact through lack of accepted boundaries, administrative machinery, political base, power to tax, and by the reluctance of provincial governments to transfer authority to the regional level. Furthermore, the strong identification of lay hospital boards and medical staff with their own hospitals and their desire for preeminence and self-sufficiency have impeded cooperative planning and differentiation of the roles of the various hospitals within a district, and have made it difficult to rationalize general and specialized services on a regional basis. The incorporation of independently administered fragments of the health service system into a coordinated regionalized machinery remains a stubborn problem. It might have been much less difficult if the initial approach to health programming had been comprehensive rather than categorical, with fiscal support emphasizing hospital construction and insurance.

Cost containment remains the overriding problem for government. The cost of health services is now well over 7 per cent of the gross national product, and the increasing cost rate is strikingly similar to that experienced in the United States. In the short run, cost containment is linked to more effective use of such resources as hospital beds and health personnel, but in the long run will be dependent upon adoption of a different approach to the maintenance of health.

A Canadian government study, based on the remarkably complete data that have been available since the advent of universal health insurance, has shown that the principal causes of death of Canadians aged five to thirty-five have been, in this order: motor vehicle accidents; other accidents; and suicide. These deaths are not preventable by medical means; they result from human foibles: carelessness, impaired driving, self-imposed risks, despair. From age thirty-five to seventy-five the top killers are cardiovascular ailments, lung cancer, and such other respiratory ailments as emphysema. Again the causes are not easily removed by conventional medicine: they include obesity, smoking, lack of exercise, high-fat diets, stress, self-imposed risks. Apart from fatalities, the records of illness requiring hospitalization put the finger, first, on cardiovascular conditions; second, on fractures and burns resulting from accidents; and third, on mental illness. Mounting an attack on these disabling conditions means a change in personal motivation and lifestyle more far reaching than anything that the energy crisis has faced us with to date. The interwoven factors of environmental and human health will be a major issue for the balance of this century, and perhaps beyond, and most of the factors involved are outside the conventional system for delivering health services.

The experience in Canada illustrates a piecemeal approach to the establishment of a system of health services. Funding mechanisms were established first for hospitals and later for medical care without a clear picture of the ultimate system of health care delivery. Resources have been applied generously to health services without too much consideration for their impact on health outcome. The flow of funds has been sustained and accelerated by the momentum of the existing systems of expenditure rather than on the basis of priorities or needs. Health services have now pushed themselves up against a firm expenditure ceiling but, at the same time that government is trying to restrain the increase in expenditures, it is faced with the problem of remodeling the system of health services, its organization, health manpower, and its balance of support from institutional and community resources. Furthermore, there is a broader and much more serious appreciation of the distinction between management of disease and maintenance of health, and a realization that such goals as health maintenance and prevention of disability may only be subjected to marginal influence through the delivery of conventional health services.

In attempting to plan for health needs and evaluate the cost and effectiveness of health services, the lack of trained personnel and the lack of a disciplined approach to the collection and analysis of information have been a serious handicap. The profusion of data collected as part of the hospital and health insurance system is of limited use since its primary purpose was to monitor costs and charges, not health. A number of important projects are now under way to evaluate specific elements of the health care system, for example, hospital care utilization, medical care utilization, quality of care, the use of nurse practitioners in primary care, screening procedures, patient compliance with therapeutic regimens, and so forth. This information will be more useful in assessing various aspects of the health care system, but all too little has been available at a time when it could have been invaluable in planning the pattern of development of the health care system. The need continues, however, to be very great. To overcome inertia, counterbalance political, institutional, and professional power, and to substitute action for motion, we need good information about health and services collected in a way that relates to the problems to be solved and to be analyzed with intelligence and integrity. This information is a valuable base for setting the general direction of health services but an indispensable element in quantitating and timing future changes. The information can also play a critical role in influencing providers to accept changes in the pattern of delivery of health care for rational rather than political and financial reasons. It is also extremely important for the evaluation of the benefits of costly innovations to the system.

The data and analytic capacity of any system are of relatively limited use if the information developed is in filing cabinets and task force reports, and if the analytic capacity is in the back rooms or on ad hoc commissions. These resources need to be at the operating level, both in planning and in the execution of policy. It is not my contention that all important jobs in the health service arena should be filled by epidemiologists and biostatisticians, but that individuals who perform these tasks should be sensitized to and informed of technical and conceptional approaches necessary to turn data into information and have a background of training and experience to apply these skills automatically in their regular work.

Similarly, epidemiologists and biostatisticians in the educational centers can have relatively little impact if they remain isolated in their own disciplinary compounds: schools of public health or departments of preventive medicine. All of our health professions need to be sensitized to the objectives and problems of the health services system and to appreciate the potential and the limitations of our data collection and analytic techniques in the hope that, when they are in practice, they will be more sensitive to the overall objectives of the health service system, and more open to accept rational evidence of need for change.

Our efforts in this regard have been limited to date. The primary problem has been lack of personnel trained in this field. Infectious disease epidemiology was not well established in Canada, and until recently there have been relatively few opportunities for postgraduate training in clinically oriented epidemiology. The amount of health services research carried out has been small in relation to biomedical research. In the past few years, however, there has been a rapid surge of interest in quality of care, health indices, and the epidemiology of health, and a growing band of clinicians doing epidemiological studies. At the same time, more economists, behavioral scientists, and scientists from other disciplines have become involved in the evaluation of health care. There has been a revival of interest in preventive medicine and health services research in our university centers and teaching hospitals. Similarly, at the regional and central levels of organization of health services, epidemiological and biostatistical studies of health and medical care services are increasingly recognized as an indispensable component of the management and planning of a health services system. The need for trained personnel far exceeds supply in spite of special measures adopted in 1970 under the new National Health Grant Act. The response in training purebred career epidemiologists will, of necessity, be slow because of the long lead-time for establishment of training programs and long transit time for the trainee. Mechanisms are required to meet the immediate manpower needs and to this end short-term training has been made available in Canada to administrators and health professionals to "retread" them for this role.

If we had it to do over again, a significantly larger investment in the development of personnel with epidemiological skills and in the promotion of health services research should have been made at a very early stage in the sequence of development of publicly administered and supported health services in Canada. It would have paid handsome dividends, I am sure, in terms of the effectiveness and economy of the services and their appropriateness to local needs. These disciplines assume even greater importance as we attempt to influence health through the modification of human behavior, life styles, and the environment.

2

THOMAS MCKEOWN, M.D.

REFLECTIONS ON HEALTH
AND HEALTH SERVICES
POLICIES IN GREAT BRITAIN

In Britain the public medical services evolved in the hundred years which preceded the introduction of the National Health Service. As in other countries, they were focused initially on the problems of communicable disease, attacked by environmental measures and the provision of clinical services, including hospitals, for infectious patients. At the beginning of this century responsibility was extended into the field of personal health by the introduction of school and, later, maternal and child health and welfare services. In 1911 the first substantial commitment was made for therapeutic services by the National Health Insurance Act. Finally, in 1948, under the National Health Service public responsibility was accepted for all health services. They were financed mainly from general taxation.

Critics of the NHS sometimes claimed that it radically changed the traditional pattern of medical services. It would be more accurate to say that it adopted with only minor modifications the framework of services which had evolved in the previous century. The inevitable reduction of the amount of private practice and the transfer of responsibility for hospitals from local authorities were important changes. But general practice continued as before; hospital and consultant services were administered on the regional basis which developed during the Second World War; and the traditional public health services were left with local government. It would probably be agreed that the most tangible achievement of the service was to make medical care available to everyone and to remove the burden of direct payment from the large number of people who could ill afford it. In addition to this positive achievement it should be said that many of the fears expressed about the public service proved to be groundless. It did not victimize doctors or public; it did not stifle initiative; it did not disturb the relationship between doctor and patient. The limitations were of a subtler kind, rooted in the tradition of the country's organization of health services. From an administrative viewpoint, perhaps the most important limitation was that while the NHS was administered centrally by a single government department, local and regional responsibilities were divided between three bodies. Hence there was no single authority with the duty and power to plan comprehensively, making the best use of resources according to a well-judged scheme of priorities; moreover, the framework of services divided hospital from domiciliary care and preventive from therapeutic medicine. Inevitably there were deficiencies, particularly in the domiciliary and community services, and in the case of the elderly, the disabled, the mentally ill, and the mentally handicapped. There were also duplications, for example, in obstetric and child health services which were divided between local authorities, general practitioners, and hospitals.

In 1974 the NHS was revised in the light of the experience of a quarter of a century. The main aim of the revision was the local and regional unification of responsibility for personal medical services. For reasons which need not be discussed here it was decided not to place the unified services under local government, and they have been assigned to new regional, area, and district health authorities. It should be recognized that the 1974 revision of the NHS was essentially administrative. It created a new framework within which the problems confronting health services can be tackled more effectively, but it did not resolve these problems. That is to say that unification of local and regional services should be seen as a necessary, rather than as a sufficient condition for future improvements; the major questions which confront health services everywhere still have to be answered. The present time is particularly suitable for an attack on these issues, for we are beginning to have a clearer picture of the major influences on health. Insight is coming from several directions: from analysis and interpretation of reasons for past improvements in health; from more critical appraisal of laboratory medicine and its contribution to control of disease; and from population (i.e., epidemiological) investigations of human biology and disease. From these and other approaches it is becoming clear that man's health is determined mainly by his behavior and by the character of the environment in which he is placed. Indeed the requirements for human health can be stated simply. Those fortunate enough to be born free of significant congenital disease or disability will remain well if three basic needs are met: they must be adequately fed; they must be protected from a wide range of hazards in the physical environment; and they must not depart radically from the pattern of personal behavior under which man evolved, for example by smoking, overeating, or sedentary living.

If this interpretation is essentially correct it follows that there is need for substantial revision of health services. The medical services of today are the result of more than a century (three centuries in the case of hospitals) of unplanned development which reflects both the predominant interest in the diagnosis and treatment of acute illness and the relative lack of concern for population measures and the provision of care. Contraceptive advice is only reluctantly accepted as an obligation of health services; whether to use financial subsidies to make food available to everyone and to influence the kinds of foods that are bought, is considered to be an economic rather than a medical question; and the control of the physical environment and modification of personal behavior are regarded as subjects of marginal interest which can be relegated to ancillary staff or even removed altogether from medical concern. But perhaps the most serious effect of the traditional approach to health services is that having overestimated the contribution of immunization and therapy, it has neglected the large classes of patients, particularly the congenitally handicapped, the psychiatric, and the geriatric, who require continuous care but appear to offer little scope for the predominant preoccupations of diagnosis and treatment.

Although the United Kingdom is only at the beginning of the required revision of services, some important steps have already been taken. For example, the present concept of the District General Hospital provides a much more satisfactory basis for hospital planning, particularly for patients needing rehabilitation and prolonged care, than the fragmented hospital system which has existed until now. The emphasis on community care, in preference to hospital care, represents a considerable advance on both humanitarian and economic grounds. The approach currently adopted to screening illustrates the more critical attack that will no doubt be needed in the development of national policies in many other fields. It may be of interest to describe briefly the approach to screening. The development of cervical cytology illustrates the way in which services have hitherto been developed, without critical evaluation. Once services are offered generally, public expectations are aroused, technicians are trained, medical staff develop strong personal commitments and it becomes impossible to modify or eliminate the service should later evidence suggest that either is desirable. During the past seven years an attempt has been made to achieve control over the introduction of screening policies. There is a screening subcommittee which reviews the evidence in respect to screening procedures, and advises the Department of Health and Social Security of England, Wales, and Scotland whether a national service can be recommended, and if not, what steps should be taken to acquire further evidence or experience. In the case of screening for breast cancer this led to establishment of a working group composed of representatives of the Government Health Departments and Universities—surgeons, radiologists, epidemiologists, and administrators. In this way it has been possible to control the development of screening services, and to initiate inquiries in respect to some of the outstanding questions: the natural history of the disease; public response to the offer of services; risks of radiation; improved methods of diagnosis; and the assessment of costs and benefits. The problems confronting policy-makers concerned with the delivery of health services such as screening are at least as complex as those raised some years ago by vaccination for poliomyelitis. They are much less well recognized.

The contribution which epidemiologists can make to a more critical approach to health services is very considerable. Many of the problems involve the collection and analysis of population data, biological, economic, and administrative, for which the epidemiologist is equipped by experience and training. At the same time it should not be forgotten that many of the problems confronting health services cannot be resolved solely, or sometimes mainly, by epidemiological evidence, but require consideration of laboratory, clinical, financial, and other data. The position is in some respects analogous to that in industry, where the information provided by scientists is not of itself a sufficient basis for decision. The problem in applying epidemiological experience to health services is not so much the production of large numbers of technical experts; it is the development of competent scientists who are in close touch with the problems confronting the administrators.

II

EPIDEMIOLOGY, HEALTH STATISTICS, AND THE ALLOCATION OF HEALTH RESOURCES AND FACILITIES

3

DONALD O. ANDERSON, M.D.

CANADA:
EPIDEMIOLOGY
IN THE PLANNING PROCESS
IN BRITISH COLUMBIA:
DESCRIPTION
OF AN EXPERIENCE
WITH A NEW MODEL

The Context

All of Canada, and its federated provinces, have enacted major social legislation to improve the health and well-being of citizens, and to redistribute Canada's economic resources in such a manner as to deal with the consequences of regional disparity (1). The success or failure of Canada's confederation ultimately will be judged through the success or failure of social legislation such as medicare, hospital insurance, the Canada Pension Plan, and others. Behind the continuing national debate on all social programs, planning structures, research and evaluative systems, the developmental and demonstration activities build up the evidence which ultimately determines the next stage in Canada's social evolution. The context is a planning process without a formal planning infrastructure. But for Canadians planning is politicized and inherent in its parliamentary form of government.

There are signs that this is changing and an infrastructure is emerging. Logic requires that both Canada as a whole and each province individually set up mechanisms which examine the success of these investments, and that evaluations should be systemwide. Canadian critics have repeatedly stressed the need for a systems approach to health care planning (2): behind this cliché is the awareness that social legislation of all types affects health and that compartmentalization of planning at the level of a single department or division in one level of government is costly and disruptive to our overall social development. The systems approach may not become the established norm in our federal system but in one way or another the planning process is now established and already is assisting provincial and federal decision-makers to select from a wide range of options those most appropriate in terms of their perception of social requirements. Because appropriateness expresses a response to some sense of need, rational planning is increasingly dependent for its success upon the content and strategies of epidemiology which measure need.

The importance of the epidemiological content of health planning has been emphasized by a Working Document recently tabled in the House of Commons by the Honorable Marc Lalonde, Minister of National Health and Welfare. In this document, *A New Perspective on the Health of Canadians* (3), a reconsideration of health planning strategies is proposed. Four components of the "health field" have been identified by a review of hospital and total morbidity in Canada. By use of such relatively simple statistics as age-specific rates and life years lost (4), the health-related activities of the Federal Government have been categorized into four components: *human biology, environment, life style, and health services.* Federal health policy and federal/provincial cost-sharing arrangements (for in Canada health is primarily a provincial responsibility) can be based upon program objectives arising out of the needs and gaps that are evident from our rich medical care data base. The establishment of these objectives and the evaluation of their attainment will require the full participation of epidemiologists in health planning. Specifically, and amongst other recommendations, this federal working paper proposes a regular national health survey, the development of health status indicators, the identification of high-risk segments of the population, the improvement and better use of the national data banks, and a research emphasis upon diseases of national concern and population life style. It would seem that epidemiological research has a sound future because of its essential contribution to the scientific basis for health planning.

The context for this projected systematic use of epidemiology should however be a sound and well-accepted science policy. Canada is still searching for consensus about how to allocate its increasingly scarce human and material resources to research and development activities (5). Repatriation of research and development activities from foreign control will entail increased Canadian investment in industrial and technological R and D activities. Research into the means of increasing and sustaining health appears to be competitive with other possible investments under this action-oriented science policy. It is precisely in this arena of controversy and national self-discovery that epidemiology struggles for funds and encouragement despite its obvious calling. Because it is a discipline usually located in medical schools, it suffers from budget cutbacks; because it is practiced in the community it is hurt badly when government expenditures are cut; because it is multiprofessional it frequently lacks committed advocates; because it is preeminently scientific it is forever struggling with the basic, clinical and social scientists for a share of the limited resources. It requires a clear commitment and sponsorship from the planning structures. The cost is too great to permit epidemiology training and employment to falter by default.

The struggle is intensified at the provincial level, for Canadian confederation assigns to the provinces, by default, the responsibility for the health of citizens. The development of a program of research in epidemiology is a rare thing for a Canadian province, and few provinces have developed a general policy for allocation of resources to research and development. Yet, in many provinces either health planning councils, cabinet subcommittees, or other structures within the Ministry of Health are being created (6). The structures vary, but each seems to emphasize a consultative role to high levels of political decision-making based upon the careful review of statistics derived partly from the health plan data bases and partly from special studies. In the Province of British Columbia an academic department, the Department of Health Care and Epidemiology (7) in the Faculty of Medicine, and an administrative division, the Division of Health Services Research and Development (8) in the multischooled Health Sciences Centre, have served several governments in a research support and advisory role and continue to explore ways of integrating epidemiological research with health planning. The relationship between these two units which have epidemiological responsibilities is shown in Figure 3–1. The activities of these structures and the research careers of their epidemiologists are the subject of this paper.

The Nature of Epidemiology in the Planning Process

However defined, epidemiology implies methods and strategies used to identify and study that which determines the level and distribution of health and disease in the community. The principal strategies are descriptive, analytic and experimental—similar to those used in any quantitative science, but their employment is predicated upon a value—the

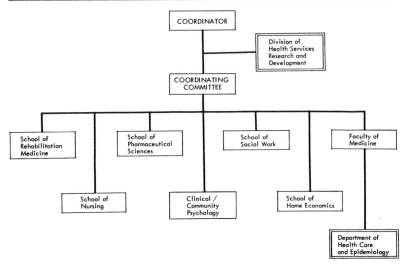

Figure 3–1. Coordination of Health Sciences Programs at the University of British Columbia and the Location of the Two Epidemiological Units.

importance of the control of disease and of the recovery or maintenance of health. All of the social sciences use similar techniques if they are numerate, and examine the probability of events under rules based on statistics and particularly sampling theory. The boundaries might appear to be fuzzy and more outlined by discipline-specific jargon than by intrinsically distinct approaches: This is especially the case in that component of medical sociology which Straus (9) called "Sociology *in* Medicine" rather than "Sociology *of* Medicine." Historically there are common roots between sociology and epidemiology and territorial disputes seem pointless (10). Epidemiology can be said to be carried out by anyone from such diverse fields as medicine, nursing, economics, sociology, psychology, and engineering, if health and disease are viewed as the dependent variable of the study and if the underlying model is causative, stressing appropriate interventions in the web of causation.

Ultimately, epidemiology examines the occurrence of events in populations at risk (11). Thus, it provides important information to the planner about targets, impacts, and benefits. There is a tendency, however, for epidemiologists to study common conditions, the diseases of prevalence. The techniques are broad enough, nevertheless, to permit useful decision-generating studies of less common conditions which fit within planning priorities. Epidemiology can be responsive to planning needs and exquisite studies can be mounted to examine various options of cause or intervention (12). This kind of analytic or experimental study is particularly rewarding in epidemiology and involves careful research design. Some examples illustrating current approaches and programs are discussed in the following (13).

EXAMPLE 1. The Department of Health Care and Epidemiology at the University of British Columbia is involved for the Provincial Government and the National Cancer Institute in the design and conduct of two such analytic studies of screening of females for malignancy. The extensive and impressive, but controversial, cervical cytology program in British Columbia (14) is finally being evaluated through a cohort study of 122,000 women: The B.C. program has been severely criticized by Knox and Doll (15) and the analysis of the natural history of cervical carcinoma and the exploration of factors other than screening is finally under way. But British Columbia is now sensitive to the cost and backlash from too precipitous an introduction of a screening program; therefore the Department is currently designing for the province a breast cancer screening project to be conducted before the program is offered to all women. The design specifically attempts to deal with methodological problems in other studies. Both studies have planning importance, and are being planned or undertaken in a way that answers planning questions which will be forthcoming; the breast cancer screening program randomized trial, however, is still being debated at the political level on ethical grounds, and may be further delayed.

EXAMPLE 2. Even a routine unsolicited epidemiological research project, if well done, may lead to a new program. In 1965 a private society established a family planning clinic in Vancouver. A review of the characteristics of users and the general Vancouver population led an epidemiologist in the Department of Health Care and Epidemiology to identify segments of the population who did not have access to birth control information and to undertake a comprehensive three-year study, the first in Canada funded by federal grants to compare matched clinic clients with general population controls, and to assess physicians' attitudes. This study reported that half of the physicians were unwilling to give contraceptive advice to single women and that many women feel they could not discuss the subject with their family physician (16). The Federal Government accepted the findings and implications and engaged the researcher for a four month consultation which led to the creation of a new federal government division in the Department of National

*Health and Welfare, the Division of Family Planning, which now pro-
motes educational programs, encourages the establishment of clinics,
and funds demographic research projects.*

The medical model of causation and disease intervention, however, is
both the strength and weakness of epidemiology. Since health planning
involves not only an examination of those factors which influence the
levels of health (not of disease) in a population, but also the cost-benefit
of different strategies and interventions, it is clear that epidemiology
cannot by itself claim to be the sole adviser or determinant either of
government policy or of the breadth and depth of new programs. The
planning system frequently requires a mixture of research personnel—of
epidemiologists, for instance, to examine outcomes, and of other social
scientists to examine process.

*EXAMPLE 3. For example, in 1974 the Minister of Health of British
Columbia pledged to the citizens a children's dental health program.
But which type should be designed? The minister created a special committee which included not only the expected admixture of dentists,
dental hygienists, and certified dental assistants, but also two economists, an epidemiologist, two specialists in preventive dentistry and a
professor from the Dental School. Rather than ask this group to negotiate an acceptable program somewhere between the poles of a public
and a private system, the minister requested that the group advise him
of the options and associated costs of feasible publicly financed programs for providing dental care for children taking into account the
need, geographic factors, the kinds and numbers of personnel required
and their training costs, and the impact each proposed program would
have upon adult dental health. On the basis of dental epidemiological
studies which had been carried out over a number of years, it was possible to work out dental needs; through an analysis of the use of dental
services by children enrolled in prepaid dental insurance, the utilization
rates and range of services were identified. Task analyses led to the design of new career options for dental auxiliaries and a ladder structure
providing upward mobility was designed and costed with Department
of Education officials. The economists, using a mathematical model, examined the best staff mix, scheduling patterns and procedural mix for
each option and the costs involved. The career life of auxiliaries was
determined from a special survey, and the intra and interprovincial
migration of dental personnel was studied from ten years of data in the
manpower data bank of the Division of Health Services Research and
Development. The report (17) presents the minister with the answer to
his original questions: two public and two private dental care programs*

for children aged three to seventeen, the costs, manpower, and impact. The next level of decision-making is political.

This example indicates that epidemiology has a very special role at the beginnin͜g of an analysis in defining need and in evaluating the success and impact of the program; however, the study was multidisciplinary throughout. Such interdisciplinary interaction is a traumatic experience because of the different conceptual models used by each discipline. While some argue that the result will be born out of the "lowest common denominator" consensus (18), the task orientation and clear challenge of influencing policy, coupled with the seniority of the members of the research consortium and their quantitative interests, in fact carried the study to the point of presenting the most senior decision-maker with well-studied options in cost-benefit terms.

Epidemiology in the planning process also plays the role of "conscience," a role also claimed by departments of preventive medicine in faculties of medicine. This role is particularly clear in government departments where the epidemiologist often is placed in a position of working with a program which is not otherwise easy to categorize and allocate to a division. A competent and creative epidemiologist can rise to this situation. Two illustrations will suffice:

EXAMPLE 4. The provincial epidemiologist was placed on a committee to examine the kinds of community care facilities and programs which should be developed. The lack of sound statistics was apparent, and a classification system of care facilities was nonexistent. An orderly registration procedure, a classification system (19) and a computer-based file system were developed; recently statistics on the numbers of beds and places in these facilities by category and regional district have been released to assist regional authorities in assessing gaps, deficiencies, and priorities.

Not all action is as rapid as the previous example and a provincial epidemiologist must maintain a vision and a long-range perspective about what is needed.

EXAMPLE 5. A decade ago after a disagreement about areas of responsibility between the Superintendent of Motor Vehicles for the province and the medical profession, the British Columbia Medical Association agreed that a medical report form would be completed on aged and medically disabled drivers. The provincial epidemiologist became consultant to this activity and a data base was established linking motor vehicle accident and violation reports with medical reports. Finally, after

ten years of data collection a compulsory provincial automobile insur-
ance system has been established and questions are now being asked
of the data which will improve the assessment of accident risk.

Applications and Techniques

In the simplified model of *need-demand-utilization-outcome* which un-
derlies most epidemiological research, epidemiology offers techniques
which define and measure needs and outcomes. Epidemiological literature is replete with concerns about definition of need—whether self-
perceived or on the basis of reproducible criteria, and the contribution
of an academic department or division of epidemiology is obvious and
too well known to require further elaboration here. Virtually every university, province, or state is engaged in descriptive and analytic studies
of the effect of environmental and life-style factors on health. The product of these studies is not limited to theoretical knowledge but to such
practical matters as threshold values, tolerance levels, and program
priorities. Our Department of Health Care and Epidemiology is especially involved in studies of air quality and health with emphasis upon
two key industries—the pulp and paper industry and the mining and
smelting industries. These studies, through advisory committees, grant-
ing mechanisms and often joint participation, are capable of practical
evaluation and policy implication: The program of research in the academic department deliberately responds to questions of importance to
policy-makers; such may be the result of funding mechanisms, but,
nonetheless, the researchers invariably serve to assist government officials both in interpretation and in the design of programs. The warm
and trusting relationship between the government and the department
has been won through twenty-five years of service to planners and is
structurally facilitated by joint appointments and rapid consultations. It
is a structural tribute to the government officials who have encouraged
the growth of epidemiology and planning at the university.

EXAMPLE 6. A specific illustration of this relationship is the action which
the Province took in 1973 when the use of herbicides and pesticides in
the forests and cattle ranches of British Columbia became a matter of
public concern, and a popular clamor arose to have the substances
banned from use. The Provincial Government responded by appointing
a three-man Royal Commission to inquire into the use of pesticides and
herbicides and into the control of animal and pest species. The commis-
sioners were the Head of the Department of Health Care and Epidemi-
ology at the University of British Columbia, a food scientist, and a pub-

lic health engineer with experience in epidemiology. Epidemiological strategies and evidence were employed to establish causal relationships between pesticide and herbicide use and damage reported in public hearings and cited by expert witnesses.

The provincial data base system draws upon the services of epidemiologists both in planning and exploitation. Canada's health care system is hard on Canada's forests, and the paper and computer-based management and accounting systems for medical and hospital services provide much potential research material.

EXAMPLE 7. The Division of Health Services Research and Development at the University of British Columbia receives from government and other agencies the following magnetic tapes of data for B.C.:

details of all patient separations from acute and extended care hospitals;

details of all day surgery performed in acute care hospitals;

registration data on community care facilities;

profiles of physicians, based upon billings to the Medical Services Commission, giving demographic information, services, and charges.

These data are not easy to use for they do not lend themselves directly to traditional epidemiological strategies of analysis. Following an innovative study of different forms of health care delivery in Saskatchewan (20) in 1969 using similar data tapes, the Division of Health Services Research and Development has started on an extensive program of research in British Columbia. Changes in the reporting forms have been proposed and accepted; special attention is being given to diagnosis encoding, in conjunction with Statistics Canada. And the data base, located at a major provincial university, is available to bona-fide researchers who are interested not only in action-oriented studies but also in scholarly research into the occurrence and distribution of disease, and the manpower and resource components of the health care system.

There are other data bases available in British Columbia. Epidemiologists are frequently called upon to design the parameters of these data bases. A knowledge of program objectives and the epidemiological literature is indispensable for this task.

EXAMPLE 8. The geneticists, pediatricians, and statisticians associated with the Division of Vital Statistics in the Province of British Columbia have played an important role in the development of two important registers: that of handicapped children and adults (21), and of cancer. These data banks have now been established for long enough periods of time, and are of sufficient quality, so that it is possible to measure the incidence and prevalence of certain diseases and complications in the general population and in special risk groups. The register of handicapping conditions has recently been expanded to include all forms of genetic disease and has been renamed the British Columbia Health Surveillance Registry. This register has resulted in at least two epidemiological studies to examine causation of Down's syndrome (22). No space-time clustering of incidence was noted, which caused those responsible for screening by aminocentesis to rule out maternal infective disease as a criterion for inclusion in the screening. And although it appeared that Down's syndrome risk was shifting to mothers of younger age, the data base indicated that this was due to a general reduction of births to mothers now over thirty-five years of age.

The strategies of epidemiology depend increasingly upon quantitative techniques which are computer-centered. As our understanding of disease improves and the multicausal nature of disease becomes increasingly important and the subject of planned social interventions, sound and efficient data management techniques are needed. While both the Division of Health Services Research and Development and the Department of Health Care and Epidemiology use the large computer system of the University of British Columbia, both have developed in-house systems analysis and programming capability. Thus, they are often in the forefront of developmental research into new ways of displaying and analyzing the provincial data base. Because the programmers are exceedingly knowledgeable about the data tapes and the epidemiologists about the quality of the data, these units customarily conduct the special research analyses for other investigators, relieving the government research divisions and using the facilities of the university computer.

Although descriptive and analytic studies are useful to planners, proof of causation is facilitated by controlled clinical trials and experimental studies where treatment or innovation is essentially randomized. These kinds of study are particularly epidemiological and represent a principal contribution from British epidemiologists; they are less frequently carried out in Canada because planning decisions require timely and highly specific research results. Rather than causation being the issue, the demand is more for information on dosage or investment; as a result, epidemiologists turn to more complex analyses of events in the data base over a long time period. Others have called this quasi-experimental (23).

EXAMPLE 9. At the University of British Columbia an important medical care research unit has been set up in the Department of Pediatrics where experimental trials of day surgery conducted with a pediatric hospital planning agency have had considerable impact upon provincial programs and received attention across Canada (24).

The techniques of epidemiology need to be shouted from the housetops. Both the Department of Health Care and Epidemiology and the Division of Health Services Research and Development provide consultation on strategies, research design, and analyses not only to other departments and faculties, but also other community agencies. It is quite clear from rejection rates of applications for National Health Grants that a principal determinant of success or failure in funding for unsolicited research is the *quality of the research design* (25). That means essentially an examination to see if the design will permit conclusions about a cause-effect relationship in one specific situation which can be generalized to other situations. The second important determinant is the importance of the project in terms of *federal and provincial priorities*. Departments of preventive medicine and their epidemiologists are uniquely able to provide consultations in both of these areas and are heavily used at the University of British Columbia.

Administrative Settings for Epidemiological Research

Epidemiological research in British Columbia is carried out in many settings: the university, agencies, government, and institutions. Each of these models makes use of different types of epidemiological professionals, for epidemiology is in no way limited to physicians.

Successful epidemiological research may be defined in many different ways. The successful application of findings from epidemiological research remains a major goal of preventive and social medicine and thus is the raison d'être for support of epidemiological research by governments. There is a problem, however, that existing structures may interfere with communications and implementation. Epidemiologists are excellent social critics and epidemiological training programs can, by stressing analysis over synthesis, prepare mere iconoclasts rather than persons with a creative epidemiological imagination. Unsolicited research may be productive in uncovering what is called "scientific fact," but in an applied field such as social and preventive medicine, unsolicited research may present sophisticated answers to planners who have not yet formulated the appropriate questions. But that conflict is an old one that lies at the root of the controversy about all national scientific policy. Epidemiology however is by definition applied: it is truly a foundation for social action. As such, it surely ranks high in any priority system for funding. But it requires new structures that will improve its access to the decision-making process.

In fact, the application of epidemiological research in Canada would be limited if conducted by academic-based researchers acting independently of structures that could bring them into close contact with decision-makers. Canada has a long tradition of Royal Commissions, Task Groups and Working Parties which place epidemiologists onto the research support staff as well as onto the Commissions; but the mix and seniority of commissioners appears to be more relevant to the implementation of results than the rational weight of sound epidemiological evidence. It is time for new structures that permit programmatic research developed in *conjunction* with decision-makers.

Figure 3–2 shows the prototypic structure for an effective epidemiological and statistical consulting unit; in fact, this structure precisely describes the relationships of the Division of Health Services Research and Development at U.B.C. The concept involves partnership with all levels of government in sharing data, resources, and research responsibilities; it describes a central role for the university as the hub of the relationship. It requires a consortium and multiple financing but it provides the Epidemiological and Statistical (E and S) Unit with direct access to federal and provincial decision-makers on an ongoing basis (26). The university base, especially in the office of a vice-president or coordinator of health sciences, provides a unique environment in a trusted, responsible, though independent body which has a research computer, access to multiprofessional and multidisciplinary resources and student researchers. Because a university is a public body, research conducted in its facilities is rarely secret but is available to the scientific and public communities. Further, promotion and reward systems of the university discourage mediocrity. Finally, such a consortium fulfills the aspirations of the university to move out from Academe to the real world of more authentic communities.

There are, however, nine important principles which characterize the processes.and structures of such an epidemiological and statistical unit which seeks to enter into a promising relationship with planning structures:

1. *Accessible, reliable, valid and constantly updated data resources* are required. This means that all data bases of the agencies must be available and stored at the E and S Unit with full updating mechanisms in

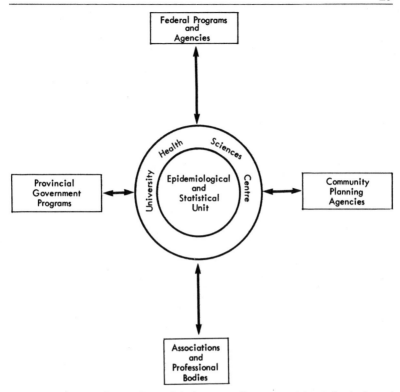

Figure 3–2. A Relational Model for an Effective Epidemiological and Statistical Unit.

operation. This concept becomes a principal element in negotiations for consultation, but the unit must be prepared to allocate resources to edit and monitor the updating and data turnover. The university may be prepared to pay the price for this in order to gain access to the data for research purposes.

2. *The controls on the use of data should be on interpretation and on confidentiality of personal identity,* rather than of a political nature. This means there must be close and honest relationships between the E and S Unit and the research units and management of each agency in order that interpretation errors are avoided and the agencies are not embarrassed by ill-conceived studies.

3. *Results must be produced in time to influence planning and programming decisions.* This involves careful scheduling and critical path
study, a clear understanding of departmental, legislative, and political
realities, and the establishment of priorities and negotiations of minimal requirements by mutual agreement of the agencies. A data processing unit controlled by the E and S Unit is essential for a rapid
response time.

4. *Results must be displayed and presented in a manner to facilitate the
maximum and rapid understanding of the material.* This means that
maps, computer graphics, time charts, as well as tables, must be used
to improve the rational process of decision-making. An E and S Unit
must continue to explore and test, with its supporting agencies, new
ways of displaying data. Surprisingly, we are increasingly discovering
that health personnel are number-bound while most other planners appear to respond to spatial displays. Discovery of methods to display
data is every bit as important as the data themselves since displays
facilitate the inductive process.

5. *The presentations must be of action-related options,* not of research
conclusions or single options. Since the initiation of the research question rests with the user agency, considerable time must be devoted to
cataloging options and testing them as an integral part of the opera-
tionalization of the research.

6. *The research activities of such a unit must be both part of a program
and responsive to priority requests from the agencies and government.*
Obviously, this is a part of good management, for the many priority requests interfere with programmatic research. Therefore the interrelationships of Figure 3–2 are essential: the contacts with federal, provincial, institutional, and manpower authorities provide early warning sig-
nals of emerging priorities and potential requests for priority research.
The manager of the E and S Unit reads the newspaper carefully as well
as minutes of meetings; from time to time he reassesses with provincial
officials the priorities and programmatics of the unit.

*EXAMPLE 10. So important is this warning system that the Division of
Health Services Research and Development staff have established a computer-based newspaper file of clippings in the health field, and each
member of the staff is responsible for a local or national paper that may
signal a change in government priorities (27).*

7. *There should be sufficient flexibility in funding* that staff can be hired
on short-term contracts to establish new data bases, conduct special

surveys and do programming that was originally unplanned for. This means that the unit should be able to charge for nonprogrammed activities.

8. *The unit must have an extraordinary sensitivity to the needs and concerns of all its client organizations while, at the same time, avoiding all secret or classified research.* This may be achieved by creating a range of reports:

Level 1. Published reports in professional journals.

Level 2. Special publication series by the unit itself which includes full interpretation as well as complete description of methodology.

Level 3. Working reports containing freestanding tables and graphics, displayed where possible in terms of options but with little or no interpretation.

Level 4. Statistical material, printouts, and other hard copy material catalogued and stored in an accessible fashion.

9. *All data,* whether stored on magnetic tape or on hard copy, *must be available for basic and graduate student research,* subject only to controls for confidentiality of personal data. This means the data should be stored at the university, tape layouts and documentation should be in the data library, and the staff be expected to assist scholars and graduate students in their use.

EXAMPLE 11. At the Division of Health Services Research and Development one of the programmers is specifically charged with this responsibility: the data base is used by students writing a thesis for the degree of Master of Science in Health Planning offered by the Department of Health Care and Epidemiology, as well as by students in doctoral programs in economics and geography.

As developed in the Division of Health Services Research and Development, all research is related to a client and conducted with an objective, a set of options, a time frame of reporting, and a reporting structure fully negotiated and agreed upon prior to the conduct of the study. Ideas, hypotheses, and requests originate from the unit itself, from its official clients, and from its university contacts, but the division does not unilaterally conduct research: rather it takes a responsive posture.

This kind of setting clearly requires a special type of epidemiologist who is favorably motivated toward the objectives and strategies of action research and of organizational-based research. Because the publications and reports do not necessarily appear in the scientific literature, and because the epidemiologist must actually think in terms of options available to decision-makers, this requires a new breed of epidemiologist—one firmly grounded in community health and committed to this style while maintaining and defending, before his colleagues, his scientific standards. Such persons are either senior with well-established careers, or junior, breaking into the field and learning, through an apprenticeship experience, both the art of judgment and risk-taking and the science of research design.

EXAMPLE 12. The relationship between the Division of Health Services Research and Development and the Department of Health Care and Epidemiology, Figure 3–1, is such that the Division provides a role model and a field or internship-type experience for students at the graduate level learning epidemiology, health planning and health care research methods from the academic department. This setting is helping to change attitudes since the director of the division is a professor in the academic department and teaches both epidemiology and health care research.

Uses of Epidemiology—a Planning Example

As a special case in point of the importance of these structural relationships, it is appropriate to review one specific planning example, the health manpower research and planning activities conducted by the Division of Health Services Research and Development.

EXAMPLE 13. Manpower planning activities are closely coordinated in British Columbia through two bodies: first, a Provincial Council, responsible for advising the Ministers of Health and Education on facilities and programs for health manpower production, has been established under new legislation creating the British Columbia Medical Centre (B.C.M.C.) (28); second, the Health Manpower Working Group has been created of senior officials in the Ministries of Health and Education to advise the Ministers on health manpower requirements for the provincial health care system. Each unit has a special research and development unit: supporting the Provincial Council is the Division of Educational Planning reporting to the council through an Education Committee of Deans and Academic Directors; supporting the Health Manpower Working Group is the Division of Health Services Research and Development at the University of British Columbia. These two units, dealing respectively with production and requirements, are linked by cross-appointments.

The Division of Health Services Research and Development also provides epidemiological and statistical services and access to the provincial data base to those planning educational and tertiary care resources. Figure 3–3 is a simplified diagram of these relationships and omits official federal/provincial and interprovincial organizational linkages. The Division of Health Services Research and Development plays an official staff role: its director is secretary of the Health Manpower Working Group, the representative of the health officials on the Education Committee of the British Columbia Medical Centre, and the provincial representative to the Federal/Provincial Health Manpower Committee, one of four continuing committees of officials advising the Council of Ministers and Conference of Deputy Ministers of Health for Canada. The Division of Health Services Research and Development is the hub of the system and the focus of all communications on health manpower development and production in the province in the manner shown in Figure 3–2; but it is also linked to planning of physical facilities.

Initially, it might appear that manpower planning is not an epidemiological activity: can epidemiology embrace the establishment of a data base on health workers, the determination of geographical and functional distribution of these workers in the province and the modeling of those forces which maintain the stock of workers? There are, however, sound reasons for relating these requirement studies to the needs of the population. For example, the Health Manpower Working Group has recommended the creation of a unified vision care service for the province, tying together optometric and ophthalmologic services based upon an assessment of needs for refractive services (29). It is currently examining the distribution of physicians and the kinds of services they provide, using this to estimate over- and underserviced areas based upon population use. Indeed, this physician study, based upon billings to the provincial medical care insurance plan, will be used to identify areas where immigrant physicians may be located under the new immigration regulations recently passed for Canada by an order-in-council (30).

The Division of Health Services Research and Development now maintains dynamic and regularly updated and official files on eighteen health worker groups which are designed to contain key identification linkage numbers in order that the various official tapes and data bases can be linked for special studies with the permission of the agencies concerned. It is an indication of the trust which the Division has won that the key linkage file for physician records, hospital services, and Medical Services Commission billings is in the possession of the division. These files are currently being broadened and updatings are being undertaken through computer-produced biographies returned by health workers at the time of their annual reregistration (31). The division releases two an-

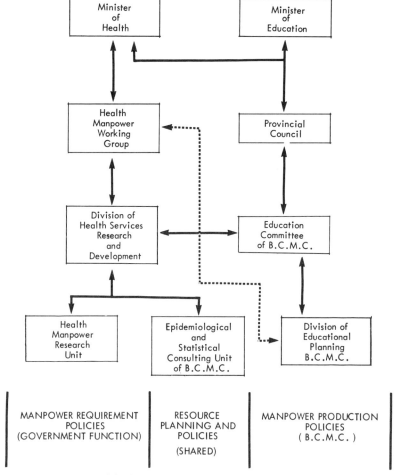

Figure 3–3. A Simplified Diagram of Health Manpower Planning Structures, British Columbia.

nual manpower reports: Output, a tabulation of all health workers currently being produced by all educational facilities in B.C. with projections for ten years, and Rollcall, a computer-produced report on each health group showing by regional hospital district the numbers, rates per 10,000 population, employer groups, jobs (or specialty), and rates of change from preceding years (32).

The principal current assignment for the division is to study and model nursing manpower requirements of all types, taking into account population needs, nursing functions and categories, positions available, vacancies, unemployment rates, and labor force participation: the objective is to advise on the location and size of new schools of nursing in community colleges which are replacing hospital schools of nursing.

EXAMPLE 14. Through its epidemiological and statistical consulting unit at the British Columbia Medical Centre the division has been active in estimating the size of tertiary care facilities for the province based upon need and utilization models. Associated with an increase in extended, intermediate, and home care programs, the acute bed requirement for the province has been lowered from 5.4 beds per 1,000 to 4.5 beds. Based upon studies of patient flow from rural areas to secondary and tertiary centers, a model has been created to identify tertiary care diseases (33) and calculate the load in the principal metropolitan area, the Greater Vancouver Regional Hospital District. Medical care tapes have been used to "mock-up" the size of a new ambulatory facility in Vancouver and determine patient load, tests generated, and procedures likely to be provided. The data bases are also being used to validate the planning requirements proposed by physician task committees designing a new teaching hospital, and to assist the Regional District in planning a new tye of community health center without beds.

The existence of data bases on staff and student addresses has permitted extrapolations of traditional research activity to study traffic and parking services for the member hospitals of the British Columbia Medical Centre (34). The provincial data bases have been used to design a provincial library network for all health institutions.

In short, epidemiological and statistical services are firmly entrenched in British Columbia in a whole range of planning services. It is an academic question where epidemiology begins and ends: the data, epidemiologic imagination and action-oriented staff have created several generations of planning and evaluation data that are being incorporated into decisions and policies. The model of Figure 3–2 is working and enshrined in legislation and regulations: an epidemiologically based planning infrastructure is a reality.

Training and Career Structure

In 1960, there were few career development programs for epidemiologists in Canada: Following a review of functions and needs (35), the

Department of National Health and Welfare created career scientist awards, called Research Positions in Epidemiology and Biometry, which were available to all medical and dental schools and government departments in Canada. More recently, training fellowships have been offered and the career awards broadened to include health services research. There appears however to be a shortage of qualified candidates. The teachers of preventive medicine in Canada have responded by creating masters and doctoral programs in epidemiology and biometry: the establishment of these programs in medical schools was hastened by an apparent increased demand for epidemiologists by universities, planning agencies, governments, special disease-related bodies such as cancer commissions, and by the demise of one of Canada's two schools of public health and the relocation of the other within a faculty of medicine. Not all of the programs however received recognition for federal funding, and there is still no consensus on where the boundaries exist between epidemiology, health services research, and planning.

Although the new degree programs are usually located in medical schools, most are multiprofessional: nurses, pharmacists, social workers, dentists, and administrators are joining physicians in the training programs. The epidemiological method has finally been retrieved from medical professional dominance. These students, on graduation, are directly moving into research positions in hospitals, community health centers, and regional planning structures. There is also a need for retraining of health professionals. The Department of Clinical Epidemiology at McMaster University has performed a major service for epidemiological training by developing a sound course of epidemiological readings, audio-visual material, problems, and a structure, the National Health Grant Health Care Evaluation Seminar (36). This package has been offered at many points in Canada and, while still under evaluation, represents a major attempt to retrain health professionals in the context of a specific research project.

In a number of provinces, and in British Columbia in particular, the government has initiated a major program of student employment during summer months. Students employed in the Ministry of Health are redeployed to many projects relating to epidemiology and evaluation of health programs. Summer learning during employment is broadening the interest in the field of epidemiology and may increase the recruitment into the field. Recognizing the fact that physician-epidemiologists may wish to receive recognition as specialists through examination by the Royal College of Physicians and Surgeons of Canada, the Royal College is contemplating changing its present Certificate in Public Health into a Certificate in Community Medicine (37). The basic training for this new field is epidemiology and biometry and the specialty will identify those physicians who deal with groups, such as in fields of public health, preventive medicine, epidemiology, community pediatrics, and community psychiatrics. There is intense interest in the draft regulations now under study both by the Council of the Royal College and the teachers of preventive medicine: the new specialty will require further expansion in the number of masters programs in epidemiology (38). A target date has been set for January 1976 to take in the first candidates for the four year specialty program.

Careers, legitimized by specialization regulations, now appear to exist in the health planning infrastructures of Canada. Health remains a social priority and the Federal and Provincial Governments, though harassed by inflation and recession, are committed to maintaining and improving the Canadian medical and hospital care system. That means proportionally a greater investment in epidemiology and health services planning relative to that in curative medicine. At least in British Columbia that appears to be the course of government action. But in British Columbia epidemiology is in the front line of health planning.

Conclusion and the Challenge

Epidemiology is too important for appropriate and adequate policy-making to be permitted to develop in an unplanned fashion according to the whims and priorities of provincial departments of postsecondary education and the universities. Cost-benefit and cost-effectiveness studies imply a need-related model and cry out for epidemiologic strategies. The establishment of a national health or medical care insurance system, as in Canada, provides the essential data for planning and evaluation and permits, under epidemiological scrutiny, the design of program changes which can select target populations of persons with high risk to diseases where effective intervention is possible (39). Because epidemiological study is the basis of all preventive programs, a shift to the prevention of environmental and life-style diseases merely intensifies the need for emphasis upon career structures and training programs in epidemiology. Essential to Canada and the United States is a major national and regional commitment to a program of epidemiological research relevant to the disease propensity of characteristics of each region and the specific health care opportunities and programs of the region. Epidemiological investigation centers must be established and charged to study diseases and social conditions relevant to the region for which they have a geographic responsibility (40). But these centers should be established according to models of organization which will bring the epidemiologists and policy-makers closer in a responsive feedback relationship. The experience gained in the planning process in British Columbia suggests this is possible. These centers are the logical field units for training epidemiologists and can bring epidemiology, in a systematic way, to address problems at the local and regional level.

Acknowledgements

The author is grateful to his many colleagues in British Columbia for permission to refer to their work. Where publications are available, these are specifically cited in the References. Further information is available on request about any specific application. Errors and misemphasis in interpretation are the author's sole responsibility.

The close relationship between the Division of Health Services Research and Development and the Department of Health Care and Epidemiology is a tribute to the creative leadership of Professor C. J. G. Mackenzie, head of the department, and Professor J. F. McCreary, Coordinator of Health Sciences at the University of British Columbia.

References

1. This issue was the subject of a federal/provincial constitutional conference; see Canada: *Income Security and Social Services,* Working Paper of the Government of Canada on the Constitution (Ottawa: Queen's Printer, 1970).

2. Science Council of Canada, *Science for Health Services,* Report Number 22 (Ottawa: Information Canada, 1974).

3. Marc Lalonde, *A New Perspective on the Health of Canadians* (Ottawa: Government of Canada, 1974). See also, H. L. Laframboise, "Health Policy. Breaking It Down into More Manageable Segments," *Canadian Medical Association Journal,* 108 (1973), 388.

4. J. M. Romeder and D. D. Gellman, *Hospital Morbidity and Total Mortality in Canada: Data for Priorities and Goals* (Ottawa: Health and Welfare Canada, 1974).

5. The concern about Canadian science policy was the subject of study by a Senate Special Committee chaired by Hon. Maurice Lamontagne. See Senate Special Committee on Science Policy, *A Science Policy for Canada* (Ottawa: Information Canada, 1972).

6. A number of provinces have recently undertaken studies of health department reorganization. The principal and controversial report in British Columbia was R. G. Foulkes, *Health Security for British Columbians,* 2 vols. (Victoria, B.C.: Minister of Health, 1973). The creation of federal, provincial, regional, and area health councils was an integral part of the Hall Royal Commission which antedated the medicare system; see Royal Commission on Health Services, *Report* (Ottawa: Queen's Printer, 1965), Vol. II, 222–36.

7. The Department of Health Care and Epidemiology in the Faculty of Medicine currently is responsible not only for teaching and research in social medicine but also for family medicine. The chairman is an epidemiologist and public health physician. Excluding the family medicine program, this teaching department presently employs an approximate staff of twelve professionals, four full time research professionals, fifteen research workers and four other support staff (total 35). In the department there are three physician epidemiologists, an epidemiological demographer, a nurse epidemiologist, three biostatisticians, and two sociologists studying disease and medical care. There are other health professionals including a public health physician and several social scientists who are engaged in nonepidemiological research. The 1974–75 budget for the social medicine program was:

University of British Columbia	$258,000
Grants	283,000
Total	$541,000

8. The Division of Health Services Research and Development is located in the Office of the Coordinator of Health Sciences of the University of British Columbia. Other divisions serving the schools and faculties of the Health Sciences Centre include Educational Support and Development, Hospital Administration, Health Systems, Business Administration, and Continuing Education in the Health Sciences. A full description is available in *A Report from the Office of the Coordinator of Health Sciences* (Vancouver, B.C.: Univ. of British Columbia, June 30, 1974). The division is headed by an epidemiologist and has a staff of eleven persons, including two research officers (statistics, education), three programmers, and two clerk editors maintaining data files. The 1974–75 budget according to source was:

Province of British Columbia	$72,000
University of British Columbia	58,000
British Columbia Medical Centre	48,000
Total	$178,000

9. Eliot Freidson, in *Professional Dominance: The Social Structure of Medical Care* (New York: Atherton Press, 1970), emphasizes this distinction, drawing upon R. Straus, "The Nature and Status of Medical Sociology," *American Sociology Review* 22 (1957), 203.

10. D. O. Anderson, "The Social Sciences and Public Health Programs— An Epidemiologist's View," *Canadian Journal of Public Health* 60 (1969), 1.

11. This emphasis upon cases/population is given by J. N. Morris, *Uses of Epidemiology*, 2nd ed. (London: E. & S. Livingstone, and Baltimore: Williams & Wilkins, 1964), p. 3.

12. Strategies to attribute causation are described in B. MacMahon and T. F. Pugh, *Epidemiology, Principles and Methods* (Boston: Little, Brown, 1970), pp. 17–46, and in M. Susser, *Causal Thinking in the Health Sciences* (New York: Oxford Univ. Press, 1973).

13. The examples, partly described in vignettes, were prepared with the assistance of John Herdman, M.D., a graduate student in the Master of Science program in Health Planning. Dr. Herdman is completing a thesis drawn from the Medical Services Commission data on practice patterns of general surgeons in nonmetropolitan British Columbia.

14. F. E. Bryans, D. A. Boyes, and H. K. Fidler, "The Influence of a Cytological Screening Program upon the Incidence of Invasive Squamous Cell Carcinoma of the Cervix in British Columbia," *American Journal of Obstetrics and Gynecology* 88 (1964), 898.

15. For example, see E. G. Knox, "Cervical Cytology: A Scrutiny of the Evidence," in *Problems and Progress in Medical Care*, ed. G. McLachlan (London: Oxford Univ. Press, 1966), pp. 279–309; H. S. Ahluwalia and R. Doll, "Mortality from Cancer of the Cervix Uteri in British Columbia and Other Parts of Canada," *British Journal of Preventive and Social Medicine* 22 (1968), 161; and L. J. Kinlen and R. Doll, "Trends in Mortality from Cancer of the Uterus in Canada and in England and Wales," *British Journal of Preventive and Social Medicine* 27 (1973), 146.

16. The studies were C. J. G. Mackenzie, "The Vancouver Family Planning Clinic. A Comparison of Two-Years' Experience," *Canadian Journal of Public Health* 59 (1958), 257; and K. E. Belanger, E. J. Bradley, and C. J. G. Mackenzie, *Social and Medical Factors of Women Attending and*

not *Attending a Family Planning Clinic* (Vancouver, B.C.: Dept. of Health Care and Epidemiology, Univ. of British Columbia, 1972).

17. The specific terms of reference set by the minister were drafted by a medical and a dental epidemiologist and clearly improved the breadth and specificity of the report. See, R. G. Evans (Chrm.), *Report, Children's Dental Health Research Project,* 2 vols. (Victoria, B.C.: Minister of Health, 1974).

18. This matter is reviewed in T. W. Bice and K. L. White, "Cross-National Comparative Research in the Utilization of Medical Services," *Medical Care* 9 (1971), 253.

19. Minister of Health, *The British Columbia Classification of Types of Health Care* (Victoria, B.C.: Dept. of Health, 1973).

20. D. O. Anderson and A. O. J. Crichton, *What Price Group Practice? A Study of Charges and Expenditures for Medical Care* (Vancouver, B.C.: Office of the Coordinator, Health Sciences Centre, 1973).

21. R. B. Lowry, J. R. Miller, A. E. Scott, and G. H. G. Renick, "Twenty Years' Experience with the Handicapped Children's Registry," International Pediatric Congress, August 1971.

22. P. A. Baird and J. R. Miller, "Some Epidemiological Aspects of Down's Syndrome in British Columbia," *British Journal of Preventive and Social Medicine* 22 (1968), 81.

23. D. T. Campbell, "Reforms as Experiments," *American Psychologist* 24 (1969), 409. See also *Quasi-Experimental Approaches: Testing Theory and Evaluating Policy,* ed. J. A. Caporaso and L. L. Roos, Jr. (Evanston, Ill.: Northwestern Univ. Press, 1973).

24. C. P. Shah, C. G. Robinson, C. Kinnis, and H. T. Davenport, "Day Care Surgery for Children: A Controlled Study of Medical Complications and Parental Attitudes," *Medical Care* 10 (1972), 437.

25. D. O. Anderson, "The Double Standard of R and D," *Canadian Journal of Public Health* 63 (1972), 317.

26. The proposal for this arrangement was made in 1973; see D. O. Anderson, "The Role of Health Sciences Centres in Health Care Re-

search" (Univ. of Calgary, Alberta: Paper presented at the opening of the Health Sciences Centre, 1973).

27. The clipping system, NEWSFILE, emphasizes key words in titles and names, legislation and organizations in the content. The report, produced quarterly, is located in the U.B.C. library where it is the principal index of health care references in newspapers.

28. Medical Centre of British Columbia Act, British Columbia, Second Session, 1973.

29. E. R. Shillington and D. O. Anderson, *Visual Care Needs and Manpower in British Columbia,* Report HSRD 73:6 (Vancouver, B.C.: Office of the Coordinator, Univ. of British Columbia, 1974).

30. Press release from the Hon. Robert Andras, Minister of Manpower and Immigration, Ottawa, Jan. 16, 1975.

31. Biographies are currently being used to update registration of pharmacists, dental hygienists, and physician interns and residents; biographical information on other groups is being collected currently and includes plans for annual updating by having reregistrants correct computer-printed biographies.

32. W. G. Manning, *Health Manpower Output of Educational Institutions, Report* HSRD 74:4 (Vancouver, B.C.: Office of the Coordinator, Univ. of British Columbia, 1974), Health Manpower Research Unit, *Rollcall-74: A Status Report of Health Personnel in the Province of British Columbia,* Report HSRD 74:5 (Vancouver, B.C.: Office of the Coordinator, Univ. of British Columbia, 1974). These data are being used in a manpower stock simulator for health manpower planning. See, for example, E. R. Shillington, *British Columbia Medical Manpower Stock Simulator I,* Report HSRD 74:2 (Vancouver, B.C.: Office of the Coordinator, Univ. of British Columbia, 1974).

33. D. O. Anderson, *The Determination of Tertiary Hospital Care Requirements, Province of British Columbia,* Report HSRD 73:3 (Vancouver, B.C.: Office of the Coordinator, Univ. of British Columbia, 1973).

34. There are six member hospitals of the British Columbia Medical Centre located in the province which are used as clinical facilities for training by the teaching institutions such as universities, community col-

leges, schools of technology, and vocational institutes in the Vancouver area.

35. D. O. Anderson, "The Epidemiologist's Dilemma, a Position Paper on the Role of Epidemiology in Canadian Research," *Canadian Medical Association Journal* 93 (1965), 1019.

36. *Methods of Health Care Evaluation,* ed. D. L. Sackett and M. S. Baskin, 2nd ed. (Hamilton, Ont.: McMaster Univ. 1973). See also, M. S. Baskin and L. Delorme, *How (on Earth) Do You Plan and Execute a Health Care Evaluation Seminar?* (Hamilton, Ont.: McMaster Univ., 1973).

37. D. O. Anderson, "Certification in Public Health—Training for Obsolescence," *Canadian Journal of Public Health* 63 (1972), 405. Reprinted in *International Journal of Epidemiology* 2 (1973), 379.

38. The new specialty in Community Medicine "draws upon the principles and techniques from the field of Social and Preventive Medicine, namely those of epidemiology and human ecology, evaluation of health services systems, organization and administration of health services, health promotion, prevention and rehabilitation" (Royal College Specialty Committee in Public Health and Preventive Medicine, 1974). The provision of training in epidemiology is a central part of any approved program.

39. D. O. Anderson, "Measurement of Use and Demand," in *Uses of Epidemiology in Planning Health Services,* ed. A. M. Davies (Belgrade: Savremena Administracija, 1973), Vol. I, 321–34.

40. In British Columbia, for example, the industrial and developmental activities of the province lend themselves to regional epidemiological investigation of a number of environmental problems such as asbestosis, kraft pulp mills, lead, motor vehicle accidents, fishing hazards, etc.

Discussion

Opening Remarks: Alan Gittlesohn, Ph.D.

Dr. Anderson has outlined what appears to be an eminently sensible approach to the involvement of epidemiology and epidemiologists in the planning, administration, and evaluation of health services. I think it is fairly clear in the United States that epidemiology as a field, with notable exceptions, of course, has given relatively little attention to this class of problems and has focused on investigations directed at etiology. Similarly, biostatisticians have tended to avoid the messy and intractable problems arising in the health services area and have been drawn into cleaner laboratory and clinical applications or into methodology and theory. It is thus possible to find a not insignificant number of biostatisticians who neglect observational data altogether because of the difficulty of drawing inferences therefrom. If epidemiology and biostatistics are to contribute to the health services field, then new approaches to turning this situation around will have to be developed. How this is to be accomplished in terms of stimulating interest, training and job placement are some of the issues which are considered in this volume.

In attempting to come to grips with medical care from an epidemiological viewpoint, one is faced at the outset with great difficulty, in many circumstances, in relating health services delivery to the health of population groups as measured in some objective sense. Until recently, most federal programs have been directed at the stimulation and promulgation of new technologies, better access, more manpower, more facilities and more services, perhaps with inadequate attention being paid to impacts on health of target groups. Both Dr. Evans and Dr. McKeown have commented that health is primarily determined by environmental, social, nutritional, and behavioral factors and, by implication, that personal medical services are of secondary importance.

In a related vein, Lewis Thomas in "The Lives of a Cell" considers the problem of technological assessment of medical services and describes three levels: the "nontechnologies" which are not amenable to evaluation in terms of capacity to alter the course of disease; the "half-way technologies" which represent efforts to compensate for disease effects after the fact; and the "effective technologies" which include certain immunizations and the appropriate use of antibiotics. In developed countries, the latter decisive approaches are relatively few in number and tend to be relatively inexpensive and easy to deliver in contrast with the former which consume, by far, the largest portion of health care expenditures. The introduction and extension of new technologies with incomplete assessment is a constant and growing concern, current examples being the rapid increase in coronary by-pass surgery and delivery by Cesarean section.

Assuming that epidemiology implies quantitative methods applied to health and disease in populations, then the potential contributions of epidemiology will be along these lines. The notion is that measurement of the medical care experience of population groups and assessment of effects on health status should be prerequisites for sound planning in the health care sector. Yet, in this country, we are only beginning to move beyond the case-by-case and the institutional focus and to develop health information systems and data bases of the type alluded to by Dr. Anderson. My own recent experience in attempts at quantification using one such data system in Vermont suggests that major difficulties exist in relating services delivered to either health needs or outcomes. Crude measurement of the utilization of services, resource allocation and expenditures for health care reveal that wide variations exist between neighboring communities of the state which we cannot relate in general to underlying disease incidence or prevalence. Examples include hospitalization rates adjusted by age ranging by a factor of two between 100 and 200 admissions per 1,000 population per year and nursing home admission rates in persons over sixty-five varying by a factor of five. The major source of variation in hospital expenditures by community turns out to be the incidence of hospitalization and not unit charges. The implication of this observation is that expenditure control through unit costs alone, as exemplified by hospital cost commissions in various states, should at least be accompanied by an examination of utilization rates. The latter can only be measured through population-type data bases.

As might be anticipated, examples of wider variability in utilization rates between hospital service areas arise when specific diagnoses and procedures are considered. Tonsillectomy, still the major cause of hospitalization in Vermont children, provides an extreme case in point. Using the cumulative risk of tonsil removal as a measure of surgical incidence, in one community two out of three children will exhibit tonsil loss by age twenty while in the four neighboring areas the loss by age twenty ranges narrowly around one in six children. Similar but somewhat less striking variability in organ loss rates is observed for the appendix, gall bladder, and uterus. By contrast, surgical admissions for clear-cut conditions where there is general agreement as to management, such as inguinal hernia and fractures, are relatively uniform in their distribution over hospital service areas of the state. The variability between areas in utilization rates for other conditions would appear to reflect uncertainty concerning efficacy and differing medical opinion concerning appropriate management.

I mention these examples to illustrate one type of contribution which the epidemiological approach might make to planning and administrative aspects of personal health care delivery. One implication is that programs to improve access to care and the distribution of manpower, facilities, and services should be accompanied by attempts to monitor the products delivered. The premise is that informed choices in the planning, administration, and evaluation of health care require knowledge of the relation between the system of care and the population being served.

Summary of General Discussion

1. Decisions that have been influenced by work or information furnished by Dr. Anderson's Division of Health Services Research and Development in British Columbia.

   a. The Lalonde White Paper essentially emerged from the work of two people in the long-range planning department who prepared a paper examining morbidity and mortality critically and innovatively and reorganized the way in which they were being considered in Canada.

b. The studies of Saskatchewan group practices led to the Saskatchewan government's agreement to global budgeting of community health centers for that particular province and led to the ability to evaluate whether budgeting had in fact changed the way in which the practices were used by the population and by the physicians and groups.

c. A new pediatric dental program is presently being designed in British Columbia, and it happens to be a program for which decisions are made at the highest level. At the present stage of program planning epidemiology has already made its contribution, presenting the minister with four basic options for a pediatric dental program and costs, taking into account the needs of the population, the geographic distribution of the population, the costs of training new kinds of health workers, the start-up time and the impact of the pediatric program upon dental health. The minister will make a final decision, and presumably epidemiology will influence this decision.

d. In the field of health manpower planning, British Columbia is moving rapidly to allocate physicians throughout the province, and decisions are being made by the Department of Health to respond to federal legislation controlling immigration of physicians. The minister has turned to the Division of Health Services Research and Development and has asked to be advised at once on the method to use in the allocation of physicians based upon a rapid assessment of the profiles of physicians currently in practice. This is a coordinated process between the epidemiologist and the government.

2. *The manner in which epidemiology is operative on the national level in Canada.*
Health in Canada is a provincial responsibility, and health policy at the national level has to be negotiated between the Federal Government and the provinces, so one must look for structures that bring the epidemiologists at the provincial level together with epidemiologists at the federal level. Such now exists in a newly created supporting structure to the Conference of Deputy Ministers of Health for Canada, in the form of four committees: Committee on Community Health, Committee on Health Manpower, Committee on Standards, and Committee on Medical and Hospital Insurance. The federal and provincial representatives on these committees include epidemiologists and researchers. The provincial representative for the Province of British Columbia on the

Federal/Provincial Health Manpower Committee, Dr. Anderson, is in a unique place as an epidemiologist, but is not the only epidemiologist on that committee. Another epidemiologist serves on the Community Health Committee. Therefore, epidemiologists have in fact infiltrated the planning infrastructures between Canada and the provinces. This means that there is epidemiological input at each of these federal-provincial meetings voiced by an official representative.

3. *The proper location and purpose of departments of preventive medicine and epidemiology.*
To follow up on the statement of Dr. Evans, that schools of public health should be dismantled, it was suggested that they might most properly be reimplanted in new locations, such as health sciences centers, where they will appeal not just to physicians but to other kinds of health workers as well. In Canada, in the United States, and in the United Kingdom training programs in epidemiology and health services research are being carried on for nurses and hospital administrators.

A Canadian training program in which this is being done offers a Master of Science degree in Health Planning. Students in this program, totaling at present about twenty-five, come from a large number of disciplines, including hospital administration, nursing, laboratory technology, and approximately one-quarter from medicine. Basing his conclusion upon these observations, Dr. Anderson offered the suggestion that epidemiology should no longer be dominated by physicians, but should be directed toward all members of the health professions.

4. *The role of epidemiology in health services planning at the ministerial level in the Province of British Columbia.*
The Department of Health Care and Epidemiology, an academic department within the University of British Columbia, and the Division of Health Services Research and Development of the Health Sciences Centre receive funds from the Ministry of Health to perform the function of defining problems and providing data preliminary to the solution of these problems. Thus one of the roles of the epidemiologist in this setting is to ask the proper question on behalf of the Minister of Health.

A case in point is the new pediatric dental program being devised in the province. The minister came into a new government with a pledge to create a pediatric dental program. Although there was money available in the province, the minister was faced with a barrage of different plans but with little information upon which to base a reasoned decision. A medical epidemiologist and a dental epidemiologist, at the invitation of the minister, advised by helping to write the letter that established a Task Committee. The letter, exceedingly specific, asked the

Task Committee to come up with a series of options and indicate the cost-benefit, taking into account the needs of the children in the province, the geographic distribution of the training programs, the start-up cost, and so forth. The question was very well framed, so that the committee had to begin with the need. There are in the Province of British Columbia continuing pediatric school health and dental health surveys providing a rich data base to be drawn upon to answer the minister's question. The time limit allotted was eight months. By drawing upon assistance from the United States and the Kilpatrick model the best mix of auxiliaries was planned, and through working closely with the Departments of Education and Continuing Education curricula were designed for different kinds of manpower to work out the training programs. The Task Committee was even able, in fact, to become involved in the negotiations with the Dental Association to examine the licensing regulations. All this came about because the question asked was not general, but was related to epidemiological concepts of the need. In the design of the question lay the answer and the design in this case involved very close contact between the minister and his advisers, who were epidemiologists.

5. *Efforts being made in Canada to attract qualified professionals to epidemiology.*

a. Funds: there are now available in Canada the National Health Grant Funds for training programs in health services research.

b. Status: epidemiology, at least in parts of western Canada, is involved in the planning process and in some aspects of the communication system, appealing to those who are interested in moving into positions of power.

c. Sound career lines: these now exist with partnerships between agencies and government, so that students are being readily employed by hospitals, planning agencies, regional planning boards, and government.

d. Medical epidemiologists: in terms of medicine, a new specialty is in the process of creation that will identify the epidemiologist who administers as a recognized specialty within the Royal College of Physicians and Surgeons. As a result there may be extra salary benefits to many for that reason.

e. Communications: across Canada the message of health care evaluation is being communicated to users, possible employers and to students. This has been admirably done by the group at McMaster, who created the Health Care Evaluation Seminar, a travel seminar that holds sessions across Canada in an attempt to present to planners and students the message of sound epidemiologically based health care evaluation. This program is stimulating both interest and applications to the training programs; it is also stimulating to some extent applications for national grants. The entire approach is rather tentative and multifocal, but doctors and allied health professionals are indeed entering the training programs and the careers offered through these programs.

4
E. G. KNOX, M.D.

GREAT BRITAIN:
A STRATEGY FOR RESEARCH
AND TRAINING IN EPIDEMIOLOGY

The main purpose of this paper is to set out both the traditional and the newer applications of the discipline of epidemiology, to examine the continuing interaction between its developing techniques and the uses to which its results are put, and to define future needs. Conclusions about the training of epidemiologists can then be drawn, and the arrangements for providing the necessary resources, that is, candidates and teachers for the job, can then be planned. The actual numbers of epidemiologists required is a separate problem and the main themes of this paper relate to the technical and material content, and the context of training, rather than numbers.

The background from which ideas will be developed is Great Britain in 1975, a country with over twenty-five years' experience with a relatively well-organized, centrally financed health service and currently experiencing the upheavals of a recent administrative reorganization of the service. Therefore, the outlets of the discipline are envisaged here in relation to relatively advanced countries where the immediate benefits of simple health care and hygiene procedures have largely been attained and which have entered the field of complex high-cost health care systems and a zone of diminishing returns. Thus, the context of health care is no longer open-ended, total expenditure cannot rise indefinitely, feasible staffing establishments (e.g., of nurses) are approaching limits and different developments within the health care field are competing with each other for resources, as well as with alternative investments in other sectors.

Extrapolations from the scene in Britain to other countries with advanced health care systems will still require care, but in many cases the necessary modifications of strategy will be questions of emphasis, and of rates and scales of investment, rather than qualitative differences. This is true at least in countries with reasonably open systems of democratic government. The political environment of course influences (and can completely determine) the pattern of health care provision, and patterns of epidemiological studies, especially those related to health care, will necessarily respond to an environment so determined. Political attitudes may affect quite directly the acceptability and applicability, and hence the utility of epidemiological studies. Professional attitudes can be even more inhibiting, and it is only recently that many doctors ceased to feel excessively threatened by scientific investigations of their activities. Until quite recently (and in some countries, still) health care research was also treated with a great suspicion by administrators, and the research workers, working from a position of enforced exclusion from administrative decision-making, often adopted an excessively critical tradition of work. At the present time, however, we may fairly say that defensive and even confrontational attitudes on the parts of the politicians, practitioners, administrators, and research workers are suffering a recession, that scientific techniques of measuring and developing the adaptation of services to needs are being developed and applied with a new confidence, and that we now have an opportunity to promote work of this kind in an imaginative, constructive, and productive manner.

Uses, Users, and Techniques of Epidemiology

Texts in epidemiology have in general been concerned with techniques and with topics rather than with outlets. Even Morris's book, *The Uses of Epidemiology* (1), served to provide a kaleidoscope view of applied studies, rather than to identify specific outlets. Pemberton's book, *Epidemiology* (2), was intentionally topic-oriented, while MacMahon and Pugh (3), Barker (4), and others structured their texts on the basis of principles and methods. It would probably not be too unacceptable if we said that these various authors avoided the crude pragmatism necessary for justifying large investments in the training and education of epidemiologists for work in service contexts. It is proposed here, by contrast, that we should, in fact, descend to this level and try to specify uses by identifying users. Strictly, this is a matter for factual inquiry, but the question will be treated for the time being as rhetorical and the answers based upon anecdote, intuition, and analysis. On that basis it is suggested that there are three main users of the results of epidemiological inquiry, namely:

other scientists, including other epidemiologists;
those providing and organizing health care services;
those providing and organizing other services influencing health.

Other Scientists

Practical health applications of epidemiological investigations frequently arise upon a complex background of interrelated studies, epidemiological and other, rather than from a single report. No single paper can be given full credit, and even when a particular study emerges as a definitive basis for action, it inevitably draws upon and refers to other work. There are many examples including the literatures on the etiologies of lung cancer, cervical cancer, cardiac ischemia, congenital malformations, hemolytic disease of the newborn, nutritional disease, and infective disease, and the study of a wide range of environmental hazards. All consist of complex cross-referenced patterns of investigations carried out in many different places over a long period of time. Indeed, the majority of reported epidemiological studies probably find their primary outlets *within* these networks. A few, only, are constructed at a moment ripe for definitive application by users other than the scientists themselves. The outputs consist of a wide range of study types, of which the main categories are observational, experimental, and methodological.

Those Providing and Organizing Health Care Services

For the purpose of this paper and of this volume, developments in health care research constitute the crucial area. This is where the major developments and changes of emphasis have occurred in the last five years and where they may be expected to continue. This has arisen partly through a relaxation of the mutual suspicions which previously existed between the organizers and investigators of health services, partly because conflicting priorities for resources have created a demand for research-based evidence and an increase in the necessary research investment, partly because academic departments have seen that their staffing problems can be answered only by constructing closer links between service and research-career pathways, partly because service careers are becoming progressively dependent upon a knowledge of and some training in health services research, and partly because the real academic challenge of the area of work has become more widely appreciated.

The changes which have occurred in Britain in the last five years should be seen as more than a phase of simple growth. There have been great changes in the attitudes of administrators to research workers, and of research workers to administrators, a change which can only be described as a change of style. These changes have been accelerated by the reorganization of the National Health Service but are probably not totally dependent upon it and it is quite likely that the movements in which we have been involved (although not alone) represent the pattern of the immediate future in many other countries.

In academic departments the main effect has been a shift toward applied work. Cherns (5) has pointed out that research activity in socially applied fields (within which we may for present purposes include health care) spans a range extending from inquiries with highly general but remotely applicable conclusions, to others which are local, topical, and possibly of short-term value, but where the intention to apply the results is immediate and constitutes an explicit part of the research plan. He calls this "action research," and if we accept his analysis much health services research lies well toward the "action" end of the spectrum. It is applied research, and it is wasted if it is not applied. Ideally, the motivation and the approach should come from those who are, in fact, faced with decision dilemmas. Even when the need for research is anticipated by the research workers themselves, it is desirable for the good design of a study to ascertain from the outset that the results can, in fact, be applied, and to elicit some assurance that they might actually be used. The people, the powers, and the administrative pathways should be identified at an early stage and there will seldom be much value in providing answers to questions which have never arisen and are unlikely to do so. Sometimes it may be possible to call into being an administrative mechanism which does not exist, but which will be shown on the basis of research to be necessary. This, however, is an admission of oblique objectives rather than an infringement of the basic principle.

One misuse of the notion of "action research" should be noted. Devotion to applications has sometimes been carried to the point where a program is all action with no research and where the virtues of involvement have been used as an excuse for failing to specify objectives or failing to produce results. It should be stated unequivocally that innovation and change without question or answer constitute an approach which is foreign to a valid philosophy of health services research. "Experiments" without research objectives are not recognized here. Health services research encompasses questions of *how* as well as questions of *what*, and the research activities may properly and intentionally interact with their environment, but there are always questions.

The change of style in the last few years has also involved the administrators. The power structure of a health service administration, and the "social" and working relationships between the research function on the one hand and the administrative and executive functions on the other, are of direct importance. They determine the content and techniques of health services research and the choice of topics which are both possible and profitable to investigate. For example, if there is no central control upon financial allocations or the deployment of resources, then there is little immediate value in research whose outlets depend upon such control. If there is no practical means of influencing the way in which practitioners behave in terms of their geographical distribution or prescribing habits, then there is no immediate value in providing data giving guidance in these respects.

The attitude of the administrators toward research is also crucial. An administration which rejects scientific studies of its own activities will in effect limit the scope of research workers to observational studies using techniques very close to those of classical observational epidemiology. They will probably be constrained chiefly to attempting the demonstration of defects in the system. On the other hand, an administration which accepts the value of research to the extent of supporting and facilitating investigations, will invoke the development and use of techniques applicable in planning and in implementation as well as in post hoc evaluation. The broadest range of research techniques will develop in a climate where research is promoted and encouraged, and where its results are used, in relation to the whole of the cybernetic cycle of evaluation, planning, and control. The methods will range far beyond simple observation and will include predictive techniques, experiments, studies, and developments of the control of implementation, the setting of operational standards and the formulation of objectives.

This, in fact, has been the direction of movement in Britain, and the techniques of health services research now extend far beyond those which the average epidemiologist might have thought necessary a short time ago. It has resulted in the requirements, first, that epidemiologists shall widen their technical range and, second, that they shall accept responsibility for supervising groups of workers with a variety of other technical and professional skills. To be specific, health care research may now be seen to include studies of:

General and local evaluations of the effectiveness of institutionally defined services such as national, regional, area, district, hospital, general-practitioner services;

General and local evaluations of the effectiveness of functionally defined services such as obstetrics, family-planning, geriatric, surveillance, accident, anesthesia, ophthalmic services;

Studies of the organization of medical and nursing practice in hospital and community;

Studies of the organization and effectiveness of screening procedures;

Investigation and development of medical information systems, including studies of content (intelligence), utilization, and engineering (e.g., computer usage, document design, system aspects);

Studies of administrative and managerial methods;

Economic assessments of services and procedures;

Comparative trials of medical and surgical procedures;

Mathematical modeling and computer simulation experiments.

The above list is abstracted from the draft research commission of the University of Birmingham Health Services Research Unit.

Those Providing and Organizing Other Services Influencing Health

An exact differentiation between these outlets and those described in the last section depends upon the exact responsibilities of the health care services. In the United Kingdom, for example, these are mainly the responsibility of the National Health Service under the administration of the Department of Health and Social Security (DHSS), although other government departments have their own special responsibilities, e.g., for industrial health, armed services, prison medical service, etc.

The provision of social services is also the responsibility of the DHSS in Great Britain, although not of the NHS. Provision of these services introduces administrative and research requirements which interdigitate with health care services. The liaison problems are well recognized and formal administrative mechanisms exist. The social services are administered through local government authorities. The local authorities are responsible also for housing policies, transport arrangements, recreational facilities, the control of atmospheric pollution, the provision of safe water and the enforcement of food hygiene. These areas are outside the field of health care, but the need for medical advice is well recognized.

It is not so clear, unfortunately, that advice is always asked, always taken, or that it is very effective advice. Although the epidemiologist can see here a large potential market for his work, it is still rather a resistant market. The same applies at the national level. Although it is becoming generally recognized that the main scope for substantial improvements in health lies in policies outside the health care services per se, there is little evidence that much has been achieved in these directions through deliberate government action. For example, major potential improvements of health are probably attainable through manipulating the quality and content of the diet available to a population, exercising constraint upon tobacco usage, the proper planning of transport and housing, and the regulation of industrial hygiene and patterns of work and employment; and yet, except in the last field, little has been done. In one sense all of these problems can be subsumed under the heading of "health education" provided that the target of this education is seen to be industrialists, architects, engineers, politicians, planners, civil servants and others in position of power, rather than the population at large. For example, the ineffectiveness of health education of the general population in controlling tobacco consumption can now be taken as demonstrated, and the main point in continuing is to create (the appearance of) a climate in which central decisions relating to taxation, or the suppression of advertising, or packaging regulations (e.g., minimum packs of 200 cigarettes) can be taken. Health education in this sense requires substantial research and raises a number of special problems. Health education has traditionally had educational objectives and has been judged in these terms; the substitution of health objectives and of evaluations based upon their achievement or nonachievement can lead to difficult problems. Additionally a target-seeking approach which redirects research toward the hand that feeds it, rather than toward the population at large, generally leads to agonizing reappraisals. It would also undoubtedly lead to a further growth of necessary techniques. Nevertheless, the basic administrative structure was, and still is, based upon a cybernetic model rather than upon a closed and inaccessible hierarchical system, and the location of research units was determined as much by these considerations as by the existence of nuclear academic centers. An effective working relationship between workers in research and administrators within a structure of this kind requires some kind of mutual bargaining position rather than the ownership of one by the other. In a layered structure like the NHS it is best if both the administrative and the research workers obtain their resources from a common source rather than that the research team shoud depend for its finance and staff establishment upon the administrative bodies whose decisions it may service.

Individual health service authorities may very well sponsor and finance the marginal costs of research carried out at their request, but the basic necessity to develop and secure the research resources on which such activities can take place should depend upon decisions and resources from a higher level. Although there is a need for administrative separation there is an equal need for operational integration. For a while this process was hindered rather than helped by a hard interpretation of a government policy that for applied research sponsored by government departments there should be a precise identification of both customers and contractors and a tightly defined contract for each research project. In time the interpretation has softened and research may now be supported either on a discrete project basis, or on a longer term program basis involving continued liaison between the contracting parties, or even on a "unit" basis with a much broader research commission. An overview of current arrangements in the United Kingdom can be obtained through perusal of two reports sponsored by Nuffield Provincial Hospitals Trust (6, 7).

At the present time the most difficult and urgent problems in the administrative development of health services research relate to career structures and job securities. This is especially so in research units where a university acts as the agent through which the research worker is employed and housed, where funds are drawn mainly from a central authority (such as DHSS), and where the staff of the unit have working affiliations with health service authorities. The staffing problems are of three kinds. The first is simply a question of the availability of high quality staff in an area of recent rapid growth; good people are hard to find. The second relates to appropriate joint appointments between the university and other authorities; there cannot be any fundamental difficulties here but the inertia is sometimes unbelievable and the goodwill of the research workers is often sorely tried. The problem, like the problem of staff shortage, is probably general throughout the world and owes more to professional ambivalence over research than to defects in administrative systems. The third problem is the most difficult and the most important; it concerns career pathways for research workers. Any unit requires a sufficient number of high-grade staff on tenured appointments, sufficient to create continuity and a critical scientific mass. At present in the United Kingdom very few workers have tenure and, when it is obtained, it has been largely limited to the university staffs (for example Directors of Units) who were already on the staff when the centers were established and who do not depend for their job security upon the contracts which they subsequently negotiate. There is little in the terms of appointments of other core staff to attract senior workers or to retain experienced ones. Even the directors, with relative security, find life difficult. They have to do a great deal of work to construct projects in order to generate people rather than, as they might prefer, have good people to generate and negotiate good projects.

There are difficulties also in reconciling administrative requirements to traditional arrangements within the university. Ratios of senior to junior workers or of academic staffs to secretarial and technical staffs may conflict with the "norms" of teaching departments, and the occasional need to appoint a research worker with special professional qualification (e.g., work study), but no university degree, may generate conflicts. It would have been surprising if difficulties had not arisen in the context of the accelerated development experienced in the United Kingdom over the last few years. Some of the problems are related specifically to the rate of change and others, no doubt, specifically to the British context. Many, however, can be seen as general, likely to recur in other places and to generate a pattern of evolution quite similar to that which we ourselves have been experiencing.

References

1. J. N. Morris, *Uses of Epidemiology* (Edinburgh: E. & S. Livingstone, and Baltimore: Williams & Wilkins, 1957, 2nd ed. 1964, 3rd ed. 1975).

2. *Epidemiology: Reports on Research and Teaching, 1962,* ed. J. Pemberton (London, New York: Oxford Univ. Press, 1963).

3. B. MacMahon and T. F. Pugh, *Epidemiology: Principles and Methods* (Boston: Little, Brown, 1970).

4. D. J. Barker and F. J. Bennett, *Practical Epidemiology* (New York: Longman, 1973).

5. A. Cherns, "Social Research and Its Diffusion," *Human Relations* 22 (1969), 209–18.

6. *Portfolio for Health,* ed. G. McLachlan (London: Oxford Univ. Press for Nuffield Provincial Hospitals Trust, 1970).

7. *Portfolio for Health 2,* ed. G. McLachlan (London: Oxford Univ. Press for Nuffield Provincial Hospitals Trust, 1973).

Discussion

Opening Remarks: Herman A. Tyroler, M.D.

In his excellent summary of epidemiologically relevant aspects of the National Health Service during the past quarter century, Professor Knox has provided us with the opportunity to profit from his insights. The points made suggest several parallels and important differences that can be drawn between United States and British experiences. A central introductory point was a discussion of the influence of the political environment on the attitude of professionals toward health care research. The problems presented by this influence appear to be quite dissimilar in Great Britain to those presented in the United States. All epidemiological inquiry has as its ultimate unit of reference a population, whether or not this is directly and immediately studied, and in the United States at present there is no one institution that has the responsibility for the provision of all health services to all identifiable individuals in free-living populations. There are obvious exceptions to this in institutional settings, such as the military, school situations, prisons, etc.

However, for total free-living populations, not only is there no one institution responsible for the provision of care, but at present it is most difficult in the United States to coordinate the collection of data which is relevant to the identification of the needs and health resources applicable to that population.

Under these circumstances, much of the epidemiological research performed here has been post hoc, observational and descriptive in nature with little immediate and discernible impact on the organization, delivery, or process of medical care. The identification of a population of individuals eligible for services, and the development of medical care responses to the needs of this population, will drastically change the climate within which health services research and epidemiological applications to it occur in this country. This will be true regardless of the particular mechanism of financing or administering the system, or delivering care.

Professor Knox emphasized the change in Great Britain in the last five years with acceptance both by academicians and administrators of action research, a most healthy and stimulating development. He points out that the power structure and the interrelationships among researchers, practitioners, and administrators are essential in the conduct of health services research, and states as an illustration, "If there is no practical means of influencing the way in which practitioners behave in terms of their geographical distribution or prescribing habits, then there is no immediate value in providing data giving guidance in these respects." We can most readily illustrate these points with examples from epidemiology and health services research in the United States:

Clinical trials of efficacy of oral hypoglycemic agents indicated their probable deleterious effect on cardiovascular mortality, but there has been no appreciable change in their use by practitioners;

Epidemiologic analyses have indicated that most currently practiced modes of multiphasic health testing have little utility, yet a paucity of trials have been initiated, and those few that have reported findings have at best suggested equivocal utility for this technique.

Neither finding has dampened enthusiasm for their nonselective use. Clinical trials of the efficacy of antihypertensive drugs have shown their clear advantage in reducing mortality in selected patients with hypertension and for some five years following the publication of these results there was little or no impact on the proportion of hypertensives under treatment in the United States. Nor does the difficulty with changing practice reside exclusively in modification of the attitudes of practitioners: trials demonstrating the equal effectiveness of nurse practitioners to physicians in certain settings have not always led to their uniform acceptance by either physician practitioners or patients.

With reference to Professor Knox's request for a cybernetic cycle of evaluating, planning, and control to extend beyond simple observation to include "predictive techniques, experiments, studies in developments of the control of implementation, and the setting of operational standards in the formulation of objectives," I would suggest that a considerable period of time for reeducation of practitioners and administrators as well as incorporation of measures of the perceived needs of services by consumers will be required before such a cycle can be instituted in the pluralistic United States health care system. Experience has been slowly accumulating in the United States at levels ranging from local community health centers, serving small but defined populations, to regional planning activities.

Professor Knox lists a broad range of studies subsumed under health care research involving multiple disciplines and technical perspectives. In addition to this excellent detail of the determinants of the provision of services, equal attention can and should be devoted to the sciences related to the demand for service, compliance of patients with medical care recommendations, and their satisfaction with it. One cannot but agree with his stress on the need to educate individuals who can influence institutions to emphasize and undertake the primary prevention of disease. In that sense, the advice given becomes truly cost-effective. However, if one further regards the health care system as one of the major environmental determinants of health in a population, then equal research attention should be addressed to an understanding of its functioning. In this context, one of the more important outcomes of the personal health services system is "care" as well as "cure."

Concerning the training of epidemiologists in the United States, two extreme positions can be identified in the health services sphere, each held by prominent and competent epidemiologists. One position argues that the training of epidemiologists should be a common enterprise, institutionally supported, independent of any specific programmatic, goal-oriented or career-oriented activity, be this health services research, a categorical disease approach such as cancer epidemiology, or the general field of environmental epidemiology. Advocates of this pedagogic philosophy argue that a solid grounding in the history and principles of epidemiology, its methods, review of successful epidemiological investigations in various fields, and criticism of ongoing studies will prepare the student for the application of epidemiological methods to any new problem he may wish to address. For example, when he ultimately addresses a new problem in the field of health services, he can readily acquire the technical knowledge and understanding of the issues unique to that field. The other position, presented here for contrast, is one which argues that the issues, technical details, and the data within the health services field are so complex, comprehensive, and idiosyncratic that only by total immersion in them during his training period can a health services epidemiologist be generated. At the University of North Carolina the training program is patterned primarily along the lines of the first position, with the additional goal of making it apparent to epidemiologists in training that detailed acquisition of knowledge of each problem under investigation is mandatory in their approach to its solution. The medical care system cannot be regarded as a black box with a population entering it and health outcomes measurements coming out. This approach cannot be pursued profitably by epidemiologists; rather, the interaction between individuals and the components of a medical care system must be made explicit if we are to understand and eventually control outcomes. The determination of statistical associations is simply not enough.

The need for health services research epidemiologists has been growing exponentially. This need has been made manifest at training institutions by requests from medical schools, governmental agencies, international as well as national at all levels, regional, state, and local, in the United States. One can predict that this is but the ascending limb of a rapid growth curve, which will come to full fruition when the planning and evaluation of health care becomes more systematically developed in the United States. Although the number of full-time teachers and practitioners of epidemiology in health services research is presently small in the United States, there is a large body of related experience, and there is potential for the expansion of research and research training efforts in this field.

In conclusion, I would like to point out that epidemiologists in the United States have come to look to their British colleagues for conceptual excellence, methodological rigor, and critical skepticism in the uses of epidemiology. Dr. Knox's presentation has reinforced this opinion and we now can add to these attributes those of flexibility and responsiveness to changing needs in the arena of health care organization and administration for practical applications of epidemiology.

Summary of General Discussion

1. *Epidemiology in the training of health administrators.*
In the United States: There is little doubt among educators and practitioners of health administration that the traditional repertoire of epidemiological techniques has a great deal to contribute. The repertoire,

however, appears to be incomplete in most epidemiological teaching in the United States, perhaps because in part it is absent from the training of the individuals, primarily physicians, who provide this training. It is very distressing to visit schools of public health and find that epidemiology's contribution to the training of administrators is minimal. To bridge this gap, the elements of the epidemiological repertoire that need to be added must be identified, and our concept of epidemiological training programs modified in order to prepare the kinds of individuals needed to fill the roles awaiting them. However, until such time as there is coordination of the planning and evaluation mechanisms for the provision of health services to large populations in the United States it will be difficult to carry out the type of teaching needed to fill these gaps.

In the United Kingdom: Perhaps one reason why there are relatively more epidemiologically trained scientists in the health services management areas in the United Kingdom (and this includes organizational theorists) is because the training of administrators includes, on the one hand, participation in epidemiological training programs, and, on the other hand, training programs for community physicians (epidemiologists) include courses on management science. In addition, health services administrators and community health physicians talk to each other and take part in each other's courses. Health services administration courses are chiefly for nonmedical administrators, while courses for community physicians are directed toward medical administration. These programs are at an early stage of development and the architects of the programs are very well aware of the need to bring together, or at least to overlap, these two patterns of training to some degree.

2. *Manpower in epidemiology.*
It is very unlikely that the United States can look forward to producing anything near the numbers of epidemiologists that are going to be needed in the near future for empirical research, planning and evaluation. A possible solution to this problem can perhaps be found by introducing epidemiological concepts and techniques into the teaching of sociology, management science, and related disciplines currently largely unaware of the existence of epidemiology as a science. A large number of disciplines are now beginning to move rapidly into the health care, health planning, and health evaluation field, and they could greatly benefit from an understanding of epidemiology.

3. *Measures taken to alleviate an acute shortage of well-trained physician epidemiologists in Canada.*
In view of the shortage of "purebred" (physician) epidemiologists and the long lead time of five to ten years to alleviate such a shortage, the

Canadian government, in 1970, adopted measures to produce "cross-bred" epidemiologists through two schemes: first, by "retreading" those in their mid-forties who were considering possible alternatives to their present careers because they had exhausted their potential to contribute to medical science through, for example, obstetrics and gynecology, or other fields, and who suddenly found the idea of participating in this area attractive. In Canada some of the best people in the field today graduated from the relatively short programs set up in this manner, for these are people who already understood the programs and problems in the health care field, and who picked up enough epidemiological perspective to work usefully with a research group, as an extension of the "purebred" epidemiologist. The second scheme is the one referred to by Dr. Anderson, the Health Care Evaluation Seminar, which went across the country into the more remote areas, influencing more people to become interested in doing this type of work locally. Again there are a number of people briefly trained who as a result of these efforts are beginning to take an interest in epidemiological projects, and who look to the "purebred" epidemiologist for guidance, so that the physician epidemiologist functions in a broader catalytic role. Both "purebred" and "crossbred" epidemiologists are greatly needed. The physician epidemiologist should be a resource unit and should be used very carefully because he is critical. At the same time an effort should be made to increase training of the "crossbred" epidemiologists, for two reasons: first, it will put adequate human resources into play in the immediate future, and second, such programs have the advantage of involving people who are already engaged in another sphere of work, be it administration, medical services or nursing services, where they have a chance of sensitizing their fellow professionals to change in ways that the epidemiologists outside that area may not recognize.

4. *The attitudes of the epidemiologist confronted with health man-power needs.*
During the last twenty years epidemiologists have sought both a professional identity for themselves and recognition from others. This has led to elitism and to the development of exclusive cliques both in the United States and in Europe. A plea for the practice of epidemiology by infiltration and for the behavioral sciences to practice epidemiology is worthwhile. It must, however, be realized that the epidemiologist cannot at the same time maintain his elitism and help others practice his discipline to improve health planning. The two are incompatible.

5

KERR L. WHITE, M.D.

OPPORTUNITIES AND NEEDS
FOR EPIDEMIOLOGY
AND HEALTH STATISTICS
IN THE UNITED STATES

The simplest definition of epidemiology is the science concerned with "that which is upon the people." The avalanche of natural and man-made grief that continues to beset the people in ever more technologically sophisticated societies suggests that either the definitions of the problems are inadequate or the designs of the solutions are inappropriate. Much of this distress is manifested by ill health and disease, and much of it is dumped at the doorstep of the health care establishment as people arrive for sorting, succor, and salvation.

Nowhere among Western industrialized countries is this social malaise being experienced with greater intensity and anxiety than in the United States. The current malfunctioning of our predominantly service economy finds some of its greatest dilemmas in allocating resources to cope with the "health" problems that are "upon the people," and, within the $115 billion annual budget for health, in allocating resources to those segments of the health care enterprise that can be expected to ameliorate, contain, or prevent these problems.

The latest national manifestation of these concerns and the major impetus for the conference on which this book is based was the enactment on January 4, 1974, of the National Health Planning and Resources

Development Act of 1974. But other recent national manifestations of these concerns have been the passage of legislation establishing the Professional Standards Review Organizations, the promulgation, in November 1974, of new utilization review regulations by the Social Security Administration, and the passage of the Health Services Research, Health Statistics, and Medical Libraries Act of 1974. There is more to come in the form of manpower legislation and national health insurance.

For all of these social experiments, epidemiology and an epidemiological perspective together with economics and an economic perspective are essential. If economics is the fundamental science for allocating monetary resources, and politics is concerned with "who gets how much for what," so epidemiology is the fundamental science for measuring needs and benefits in the health sector. If we are going to count money and costs, on the one hand, so we must be able to count benefits and value, on the other. Some things are valued more than others by different groups, and politicians and administrators cannot allocate resources sensibly and fairly without improved measures of value (see Figure 5–1).

Over the past quarter-century, the United States has experienced three largely abortive attempts to plan health services: the Hill-Burton Program built acute care hospitals to the point where the country is substantially overbedded; the Regional Medical Programs expanded the notion that exemplary subspecialty or tertiary care is a substitute for exemplary primary or general health care; and the Comprehensive Health Planning Agencies tried to negotiate the future without relevant information, fiscal control, or political "clout." For the most part, these programs floundered because they lacked a perspective based on the measurement of the perceived needs of the people to whom the beds, services, and plans were directed and whose interests they were supposed to serve. Other fiscal and epidemiological aberrations include, for example, the proliferation of categorical service programs for special needs like family planning, sickle cell anemia, and hypertension in contrast to general care; categorical payment mechanisms that cover end-stage renal disease but not the beginning stages; and cost reimbursement schemes that favor the use of more expensive resources such as hospitals and encourage elective surgery of doubtful value. Collectively, these piecemeal approaches are now perceived by the public as inequitable, wasteful, and unsatisfactory.

New mandates have been established and these bring new opportunities and challenges for allocating resources more realistically than has been the case in the United States in the past quarter-century. It is here that both history and experiences of other countries can be informative. Indeed, the political art of resource allocation is a universal phenome-

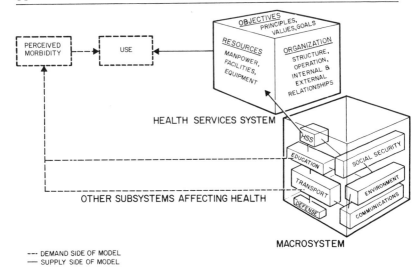

Figure 5–1. The Health Services System Within the Macrosystem of Society

From: *Health Care: An International Study,* eds. R. Kohn and K. L. White (London and New York: Oxford Univ. Press, 1976).

non without geographical or temporal boundaries; it is employed by individuals, families, states, regions, nations, and around the world as we all recognize the need for more sensible allocations of our collective and largely finite resources. From these and other pressures, not even the health care establishment is exempt.

Political arithmetic had its origins during the Italian Renaissance in Florence and Venice but its applications to health were the work of William Petty (1623–87), a physician, economist, and scientist who became Professor of Anatomy at Oxford and Vice-President of Brasenose College. His interests in biological variation extended to a concern for variation among and between populations, especially with respect to the interactions of social conditions and the health status of communities, and to these he applied quantitative methods and calculations. However, it was Petty's friendship with the London merchant-turned-accountant John Graunt (1600–1674) which resulted in the first public manifestation of political arithmetic, the latter's classic "Natural and Political Observations upon the Bills of Mortality," published in London in 1662 (1). In this epidemiological treatise Graunt showed the differential impact on death rates of variations in living and working conditions in Britain.

From these beginnings, political or social arithmetic, as it came to be called, has advanced for three hundred years. Unfortunately, these advances, important as they have been in defining the broad tasks of any health care establishment, have become increasingly divorced from both the mainstream of medicine in medical schools and from their intellectual origins in the universities. The bureaucratization of both action and knowledge has isolated epidemiology and health statistics, together with their capacity for guiding and monitoring the health enterprise and relating it to other social forces. The segregation of these disciplines in schools of public health some sixty years ago appears to have been motivated more by academic politics, institutional rivalries, and fund raising prospects than by responses to social need or scientific challenges (2). Similarly, the separation of demography and sociology from their intellectual cousins, epidemiology and health statistics, and their resultant lack of exposure to the problems of health as they arise in social milieus, constitutes an important impediment to the contributions of all four disciplines in understanding and improving the human condition and the people's health. Medicine in the United States has made some notable advances because of its links with the natural sciences, especially physics and chemistry and, to a lesser extent, human biology. But since the days of Flexner, it has done this at the cost of gross neglect of other factors that may well have a much greater influence on health and disease, and at the cost of great imbalance in the manpower and services provided to meet the needs of society in coping with its health problems. It is time to remove these barriers to achieving a balanced view of medicine's tasks and of society's needs; epidemiology and the epidemiological viewpoint are in a strong position to assist in redressing the imbalance.

If traditional medicine emphasizes the one-to-one relationship between patient and physician, certainly the central transaction in clinical medicine, there is now need to recognize the additional collective relationship between all physicians, the entire health care establishment, and all the people. This "epidemiological shift" recognizes the interest of clinicians in numerator data, that is, sick patients who seek care, and the interest of demographers and sociologists in denominator data, that is, the structure and dynamics of populations, but it goes further, for epidemiology is concerned with both parts of the fraction. The epidemiologist is concerned with relating the sick who seek care to those who are sick but do not seek or receive care; he is, indeed, concerned both with all those who are sick and all those who are at risk of becoming sick.

This larger societal viewpoint is at the heart of the epidemiologist's interest in rates and ratios, in samples, in the definition of populations, in the use of comparable terms, definitions, and classification schemes, in the application of standardization procedures that permit comparisons over time and place, and in the estimation of bias through the recognition of the influences of observer error, observer variation, institutional selection, and of the ubiquitous impact of the placebo and Hawthorne effects on most clinical transactions. Of all this the contemporary graduate of an American medical school is largely ignorant. Indeed, it is not unfair to say that he is largely nonnumerate and largely uncritical; his capacity to judge what medicine and medical science can and cannot contribute to human welfare in relationship to human needs is meager at best.

How else can we explain the rampant polypharmacy or the glut of part-time surgeons in this country? How else can we explain such phenomena as the use of national estimates of morbidity, mortality, and use of health services for planning local Regional Medical Programs without regard for the effects of sample size or the influence of local variations in the age and sex structure? How else can we explain the inability of physicians and administrators to grasp the notion that reliable estimates within acceptable confidence limits can be based on a probability (not a haphazard) sample of the population, community, or universe being studied? (Presumably, hematologists understand the difference between examining the patient's entire blood volume and examining a sample of the patient's blood!) Yet there are large numbers of physicians in positions of authority and responsibility in universities, hospitals, and health departments (especially the Department of Health, Education and Welfare), and on utilization review committees and PSRO's, who do not understand the basic concepts of a probability sample, of measures of central tendency, of biological variation, of rates, or of standardization. Nevertheless, they talk glibly of computers and systems analysis and wonder why the results are both costly and confusing. How do we explain the widespread confusion among outpatient departments and their administrators, now so deeply concerned with "ambulatory medicine," "emergency services" and "primary care," when the differences between counts of visits, diagnoses, problems, patients, cases, and persons at risk are not understood? Lacking common usage of terms, the resultant impossibility of making objective comparisons within and between institutions should not be surprising. How do we explain the current emphasis in the PSRO's on "process" measures and the detection of idiosyncratic aberrations of individual physicians and their patients, rather than on aggregated "outcome" variables based on institutional performance or the experiences of general populations? How do we explain the history of widely touted remedies, generated in the era of so-called scientific medicine, that have been shown to be useless; these include such common measures as the bland diet for peptic ulcer, bed rest for infectious hepatitis, gastric freezing, and portacaval shunts, to list a few of the more troublesome, expensive or dangerous procedures. The latest candidates for retrospective critical examination with respect to their efficacy and effectiveness are coronary artery bypass surgery, coronary care units, and EMI brain scanners. For example, at the rate that EMI scanners are being installed (140 ordered by March 1975), there will soon be a capacity for performing at least a million brain scans per year at a cost of an initial investment of about $70 million and annual operating expenditures of $300 million (3). If we use as a rough estimate of need the 16 million physician visits per year for headaches, this assumes that perhaps one in 16 physician visits for headaches is associated with a serious risk of a brain tumor. The latest available mortality figures for the United States indicate that in 1969, 6,085 persons died of malignant brain tumors and another 197 of benign tumors, or a total of less than 6,300 persons (4). The overall risk of having a brain tumor for those with headaches consulting physicians is, therefore, about one in 2,500 visits, yet we are gearing up with a highly expensive technological test as if the risk were one in 16 visits. Even if it is argued that all those with any form of diagnosed cerebrovascular disease should have it confirmed by a brain scan, there were only 530,000 persons discharged in 1971 from U.S. short-stay hospitals categorized under this ICDA diagnostic rubric, so that we will shortly have twice the necessary capacity to deal with their problems (5). By April 1976, there were over 300 brain scanners installed and perhaps as many more on order; how many do we need or can we afford? This kind of extravagant approach to resource allocation for health care makes neither clinical nor fiscal sense.

If all our new enterprises and procedures were inexpensive or benign with respect to their hazards, our concerns might be minimal. Current estimates are that at least a quarter of the $130 billion annual health care budget in the United States is wasteful, and without substantial changes both the absolute and proportional waste may be substantially higher in the future (6).

How are clinicians, administrators, and politicians to learn "statistical compassion," to use Walsh McDermott's phrase, in addition to individual compassion? How can they be given estimates of the relative costs and benefits for various services and estimates of the populations who would benefit from the postponement of death, from the reduction of disability and distress, and from the amelioration of discomfort? How can the politicians and administrators help to choose between investments in more hospital beds, more physicians, or more nonprofessional health care personnel? Should these be short-term or long-term beds? Are large hospitals to be preferred to small hospitals? Should the physicians be generalists or specialists and in what proportions, and should the other health care personnel be trained as technicians or as counsellors? And even more important, how much should be invested in the short term and how much in the long term? How much in applied science and how much in fundamental science? None of these questions is easy; the answers are political, not epidemiological, clinical, or economic. In spite of 300 years of history, epidemiology and health statistics are still young sciences, but they can contribute infinitely more conceptually, managerially, and methodologically than they have done in this country to date. Epidemiology is, in fact, based on a rather simple set of ideas and methods, but this discipline especially can contribute to a point of view that gives primacy to concerns of the public in describing their health problems and the circumstances in which these arise, and to the evaluation of the impact of the health care establishment on those problems through its manpower, resources, and services. It is by closing the cybernetic loop through evaluation that the next set of political and administrative decisions can be better informed than those that preceded them (see Figure 5–2). This was the goal of political arithmetic espoused by Petty and Graunt 300 years ago. It is at least in part the reality that epidemiology can contribute in this country, if the experiences of other countries constitute a useful guide.

Let me list a series of questions, paraphrased from Sir Douglas Black, that any administrator or politician responsible for resource allocation should address to the proponent of any procedure or service (7):

What are the aims of the procedure or service in question?

How many people, and of what kinds, are potentially eligible for help from these procedures or services?

What proportion of these people actually get help?

What kinds of people are they, and who fails to get help?

What determines who gets this help, and who does not?

Does the procedure or service do any good or make any discernible difference? To whom?

What does this procedure or service cost? How do these costs compare with those of potential substitutes?

Who pays?

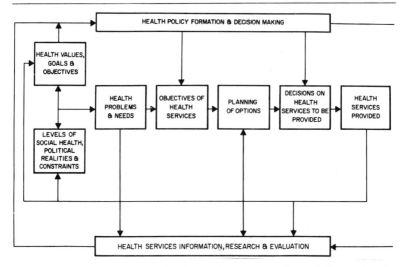

Figure 5–2. The Functions of Information, Research, and Evaluation in Health Services System Policy Formation
From: *Health Care: An International Study,* eds. R. Kohn and K. L. White (London and New York: Oxford Univ. Press, 1976).

What does the public, those served, those eligible but not served, and those ineligible, think about the procedure or service?

What impact might the procedure or service make on the demand for and effectiveness of other procedures or services?

There are six areas in which epidemiology can be a powerful force in helping decision-makers with these questions.

1. *Etiology.* The traditional search for causal agents or configurations of risk factors should be pursued vigorously but in the future perhaps it should be approached from an ecological perspective with respect to the nature of disease and its genesis. Indeed, the detection of each new agent or factor found to be necessary, if not sufficient, for the development of any recognizable ailment places us closer to ultimate prevention or cure. Epidemiology is likely to play an increasingly important role in this regard as new sources of data emerge with the development of contemporary health information systems.

2. *Efficacy.* This is concerned with establishing objectively that a new form of preventive, diagnostic, curative, or restorative intervention is more useful and beneficial than it is harmful or useless for the purposes for which it is advocated, or than the type of intervention it is designed to replace or, in fact, whether it is better than doing nothing. This is the arena of the randomized clinical trial introduced in the United Kingdom by Sir Austin Bradford Hill and in the United States by Professor Donald Mainland twenty years ago, and recently so vigorously and articulately espoused by Professor A. L. Cochrane (8). While there may be other experimental or observational designs that provide for the control of selective bias and the placebo and Hawthorne effects, the predominant instrument is certainly that of the randomized clinical trial. It should be noted that the methods for assessing the efficacy of clinical measures are also applicable to the study of administrative practices.

3. *Effectiveness.* This is concerned with measuring the extent to which an efficacious form of intervention can be shown to have been made available or applied to all those in a defined population who could benefit from it. Effectiveness studies are as concerned with those who do not use health services or receive efficacious forms of intervention as they are with those who do.

4. *Efficiency.* This is concerned with measuring the extent to which a stated level of effectiveness can be achieved with the lowest expenditures of personnel, resources, and money. One part of the equation involves monetary units or equivalents but the other half requires measures of disability levels, health status, or disease prevalence expressed in units with which epidemiologists are familiar. They are essential participants in designing and conducting such studies.

5. *Evaluation.* This is a generic term that can be applied to studies of efficacy, effectiveness, and efficiency. It requires the expression of a goal, objective, or standard that is in some sense "valued," and an assessment of the extent to which that objective or standard is achieved as a result of some form of intervention or provision of services. This is an approach to the problems of health and health care in which epidemiologists are especially suited to participate.

6. *Education.* Finally, there is education. There is not only the challenge of preparing new generations of epidemiologists but the equally great opportunity, if not the obligation, to sensitize and acquaint clinicians, administrators, and policy-makers with the epidemiological viewpoint and perspective. Epidemiologists can assist their colleagues in recogniz-

ing the need for epidemiological and statistical information in the development of any arrangement of health services that seeks to balance equity of access to care, fair shares in the distribution of resources, and responsible moderation of costs. Clinicians and administrators will have to consider the needs both of populations as well as those of individual patients. To inculcate statistical compassion in administrators and policy-makers may be as important as encouraging personal compassion in clinicians.

How many epidemiologists are needed to do all these good things in the United States? My most conservative estimate is 2,500 immediately, or one for each forty million dollars we spend annually. There should certainly be at least four or five epidemiologists for each medical school, one for each major clinical service and one for the dean's office, or 500 altogether. Each major nonuniversity hospital also needs at least one epidemiologist or 500 for the largest hospitals. If there are to be perhaps 200 Health Systems Agencies under the new planning bill and fifty State Health Planning and Development Agencies, they will each require an average of two epidemiologists or another 500 altogether. The 200 PSRO's and their related State Councils should require at least one each or another 200. The Cooperative Federal-State-Local Health Statistics System now being established probably needs 300 more epidemiologists, and state regulatory bodies, insurance carriers, hospital associations, and voluntary agencies could easily absorb another 500 for a grand total of 2,500. Based on memberships in professional organizations, there are probably no more than 500 fully trained epidemiologists and another 400 health statisticians in the country, and of this total, probably no more than 300 are physicians. These are extremely conservative estimates. If there is any thought that I exaggerate, these figures can be compared to the careful calculations made for the reorganized National Health Service in Scotland, where it is estimated that about 200 "community medicine specialists," primarily medical epidemiologists, will be needed for five million people (9). The United States, on that basis, would need 8,000 medically trained epidemiologists (apart from health statisticians) or one for every 40 physicians, a far cry from my basic estimate of 2,500 or one for every 125 physicians. The latter is only a start, but indeed a start should be made.

What can be done next? Here are six suggestions.

1. The evolution of university health sciences centers should be accelerated. The epidemiological viewpoint, including the use of contemporary health information systems, should guide the allocation of resources and the development of educational activities. Furthermore, schools of

public health should be amalgamated with medical schools; perhaps the viewpoint of the former should predominate in the councils of the university health sciences centers. The University of Toronto has set an example in this direction and American universities would do well to follow this experience carefully.

2. The United States Congress, either as a part of the Social Security provisions, the NIH appropriations, or national health insurance legislation, should provide an additional 10 per cent for all research and development grants in medicine and health services that purport to be concerned with some preventive, diagnostic, or therapeutic procedure. These funds should be used for the mandatory conduct of a randomized clinical trial or similar experimental or evaluative study to determine the efficacy or effectiveness of each new procedure developed with support from federal funds. Without such trials and evaluations, we are likely to propagate further waste, permit use of harmful procedures to co-opt scarce resources, increase the hazards to patients, and inflate the cost of care.

3. Philanthropic foundations should undertake the vigorous and generous support of departments of epidemiology and related research and training programs in selected university health sciences centers around the country. Without substantially strengthening these university departments, it is unlikely that there will be any prospect of meeting the country's needs.

4. University health sciences centers should establish or broaden the mandates of current Health Services Research and Development Centers to include support for all forms of clinical evaluation and the conduct of randomized clinical trials, so that faculty and students work and learn in a climate of critical and scientifically based skepticism with respect to all forms of clinical and administrative intervention.

5. The United States Department of Health, Education and Welfare should stimulate the employment of epidemiologists by PSRO's, Health System Agencies, and statistical units participating in the Cooperative Federal-State-Local Health Statistical System. In addition, they should see that all resource-allocating councils, committees, and other executive and advisory bodies have staff epidemiologists available to them.

6. Congressional committees should encourage those who advocate special causes, such as the one I am espousing, to present numbers and to relate costs to benefits. How can Congress appropriate resources to

meet needs without knowing who gets how much for what? It would cost perhaps $50,000 to train each epidemiologist or about $100 million to train 2,000 and $400 million to train 8,000 epidemiologists. These are paltry sums in relation to the essential contributions of epidemiologists and health statisticians and to more sensible and prudent resource allocation; they might go a long way toward reducing the $25 billion of our national health budget that we waste annually.

References

1. M. Greenwood, *Medical Statistics from Graunt to Farr* (Cambridge, England: Cambridge Univ. Press, 1948).

2. G. Williams, "Schools of Public Health: Their Doing and Undoing" (Unpublished manuscript, 1966).

3. *Wall Street Journal,* March 14, 1975.

4. United States National Center for Health Statistics, unpublished data.

5. United States National Center for Health Statistics, *Inpatient Utilization of Short-Stay Hospitals, by Diagnosis, United States* (Washington, D.C.: U.S. Dept. of Health, Education, and Welfare, Publication No. (HRA)75–1767, 1971).

6. Statement of Sydney Wolfe, M.D., Public Citizen's Health Research Group, U.S. Dept. of Health, Education, and Welfare Conference on Inflation (Washington, D.C.: [processed], Sept. 19–20, 1974).

7. D. Black, "What Should Now Be Done by Government?" Symposium No. 15, Constraints on Medicine, *Proceedings of the Royal Society of Medicine,* 67, Part 2 (1974), 1306–8.

8. A. L. Cochrane, *Effectiveness and Efficiency: Random Reflections on Health Services* (London: The Nuffield Provincial Hospitals Trust, 1972).

9. Scottish Home and Health Department, *Community Medicine in Scotland* (Edinburgh: Her Majesty's Stationery Office, 1973).

Discussion

Opening Remarks: Walter McNerney

From the point of view of the manager, I strongly agree with the following points made by Dr. White:

More epidemiological perspective is needed in the health field, and this need is immediate;

The epidemiological perspective applies conceptually to administrative practices as well as clinical practices; its use, however, has been largely ineffective in the planning of health services and other areas;

Most medical practitioners and health administrators fail to think in epidemiological terms, thus permitting and fostering the existence of an almost universal preoccupation with process rather than with outcome; in short, the entire system is tilted by economic pressures toward the expensive technological side;

Waste in our present system is indeed significant, to a point that in many areas the system could be expanded or contracted without measurable impact on morbidity or mortality. Much of this waste could be reduced by broader and more sophisticated use of epidemiological techniques and points of view.

The lack of epidemiological perspective is a function of several influences:

The whole system is excessively geared to the free choice of a physician and a one-to-one relationship with him; our psychological investment is in seeing a doctor when feeling ill, whether the condition requires it or not, and this is hardly the soil for community solutions.

Health is defined by health practitioners in excessively narrow terms, while good health is a function of numerous influences, many of which (income, housing, life style) are outside the traditional boundaries of the health care system, a sure symptom that the system in the United States is not geared to results, but rather to means.

Institutionalization of the health care field and preoccupation with the ends of the institution rather than the needs of the community to be served.

To express the institutionalization phenomenon another way, the field is captured by the technocrat: there is widespread belief that the most complex treatment is the best treatment, that equipment and specialization, rather than reason, is the best answer to community problems.

The low leverage of the health administrator in hospitals, the Department of Health, Education and Welfare, state health departments, and so forth. As a result, responsibilities tend to flow along functional and professional rather than program or project lines, and accountability is largely untested by either expenses related to goals and a budget or by accomplished versus projected results; in many instances, goals are not set forth and questions remain unasked by management because of a despair over the prospect of being able to follow through.

The entire system is on the defensive in a malpractice environment, rife with individual and class action suits. As a result, field trials and similar endeavors become improbable, conservatism in generous amounts becomes the order of the day, and treatment is geared to what is customary, whether effective or not.

The problems of middle and advanced age involve a large number of relative variables, and it is more difficult to reduce benefit to a single value for comparison of costs and priorities, requiring more skill and more money and drastically reducing the number eligible to participate.

It is important to note that the shortfall in adopting an epidemiological perspective is growing, even as costs are rising against scarce resources, and public expectations toward the health care field are growing, albeit with some skepticism. Technology is doubling every ten years, promoting more specialization and a wider gap between the instruments in service and the users of services. Reaching further back, the general environment for promoting epidemiology or any discipline other than professional practice remains weak. As in all countries, the health care market is weak, thus putting minimal pressure on the decision-maker. The problem is compounded by the fact that our political market, lacking a strong tradition, is geared to categorical programs, often piled on one another. It is an environment in which the ambivalence over demand and need frustrates epidemiology and cries for it in the same breath.

In summary, I believe that the following points should be stressed. We need more epidemiologists and more epidemiological training, to be sure, but we also need to change the health care system in the United States. A better balance must be struck between the requirements of the profession and those of the community, between process and results. This will require stronger management at the institutional and area levels; it will require an assertive national health insurance system geared against goals and providing a total system against which epidemiology can function; and it will require planning on both regional and national scales. Without these reforms, epidemiology and other elements of the health care field (health education, rehabilitation) will not come about.

An even greater consumer input is needed in order to overcome the forces of technology and institutionalization and to create a friendly environment for community questions.

Epidemiological concepts need to be incorporated by the whole management team and opportunities provided for continuing education in the field.

We need to see a greater reference to demonstrations, as opposed to specialization. The worth of epidemiology must be shown in a familiar setting: a medical center working with a state or region could be an ideal combination for such demonstrations.

Finally, there is a certain amount of outrage seen in epidemiological circles because systems are not more rational, as if decisions made in other areas were. Some of the shortfall must be accepted by the epidemiologist himself. If epidemiology aspires to be a community force as well as an institutional one, it must learn the politics of group behavior as well as the influence of group phenomena. This is learned in the field, although more could possibly be built into the curriculum, and in the last analysis it is wise to ally oneself with shrewd managers of change, able to provide the proper setting without which epidemiology will lose inevitably to the one-to-one concept of medicine.

Summary of General Discussion

1. *The difficulty of reconciling the needs of the individual patient with the perspectives provided by a population approach.*
One might ask the clinician to add to his routine inquiries questions such as, why was this patient admitted to the hospital on this particular day; why didn't he come last week or some other time; why does he come to this particular hospital at this time and what does he expect of this particular consultation? By asking these kinds of questions issues are raised such as the possibility of prevention and the possibility of alternative modes of treatment. Much more preventive medicine can be taught in those circumstances and a much greater awareness of the epidemiological distribution of diseases can be generated than by more standard means such as textbooks and lectures.

Perhaps this difficult issue can be resolved at least partially by bearing in mind the point made by Dr. McKeown, that there are at least three related but separable issues requiring the application of epidemiological data for health services planning and evaluation. These issues are questions relating to the financing of health care, to the organization and management of health care, and to the content of health care. The importance of keeping these issues separate is that they each require a different degree of value judgment, in addition to data for their solution. It is perhaps in the issues involving financing of care that the discrepancy between individual and population needs is greatest and where the most difficult value judgments have to be made. In the area of the content of health care (the efficacy, for example, of different screening, diagnostic, and therapeutic methods), there is much less discrepancy between epidemiological findings and the individual patient's needs. If it is found, for example, that patients discharged after two days following a given operation have no more complications, are satisfied and become fully functional at an earlier stage than patients discharged after ten days, there does not appear to be any reason why these findings cannot be applied to each individual patient, allowing, of course, for a few exceptional circumstances.

2. *Regionalization of health care systems.* It is important in the management of health care systems to recognize that regionalization does not exclusively entail geographical regionalization, as suggested by our European models. One can also regionalize by health care systems, in which there is an enrolled population. The contract defining the patient–system relationship for this population is not necessarily financial; it can be symbolized by a plastic card or by a verbal or written understanding. One can regionalize by enrolled groups or populations of a hundred thousand or half a million in systems that cut across geographic bailiwicks. Each of these, for example a state, could franchise or license a particular system that might have enrollees in several states. It is essential to realize that we are not locked into a geographical system of regionalization in the United States.

3. *The need for an interdisciplinary approach to health services research.* Clearly, the bulk of the issues raised by Dr. White are not medical questions at all, but questions that require education and knowledge in a variety of areas. One reason that health care systems in the United States and probably elsewhere are in their present state is that the M.D. degree has been regarded as a credential for doing all of the planning, regulating, and evaluating that has been done, even though the person with the degree has been given little or no background preparing him for such responsibilities. Simultaneously the requirement for credentials has turned away many good people with appropriate training in the several disciplines required who might have contributed to some of the tasks that have been described. Clearly one of the major needs, as several people have pointed out, is for better information collection, analysis, and utilization, but as it has also been pointed out by Dr. White, Mr. McNerney and others, need by itself will not solve the problem. Managers, planners, regulators, and evaluators are needed, and above all, a far more sophisticated consumer is greatly needed. There does not appear to be a single answer as to what institutional arrangements are best with respect to remedying the present situation educationally. It has been suggested that schools of public health be abolished. There are, no doubt, many arguments in favor of such action, but the question remains whether that alone will solve any problems. The complexity of the questions is such that the type of education being discussed here is the business of the university as a whole and of relationships between

the university and outside agencies. What is needed are new, different institutional arrangements to meet needs that are in many instances quite recent. A case in point is a new program in Health Policy and Management at the Harvard School of Public Health, a program jointly run by the School of Public Health, the Medical School, the School of Government, and the Business School. To attempt to derive all of the expertise required to run such a program from any single institution would almost surely be to settle for less than the best in a variety of disciplines. As far as research efforts are concerned, the Harvard School of Public Health has, like many others, undertaken multidisciplinary approaches. It is a long, difficult process for people to begin to speak each other's language, but it does happen. There is today extra interest on the part of wide sectors of the university and on the part of people outside of the university in such approaches, and this interest should be exploited and encouraged.

6

MAUREEN M. HENDERSON, M.D.

NEEDS AND RESOURCES FOR EPIDEMIOLOGY AND HEALTH STATISTICS IN THE UNITED STATES

This paper concerns the needs and resources for three types of professionals: physician epidemiologists, epidemiologists, and biostatisticians with the equivalent of doctoral level training. Demographers, nurses, biostatisticians, and others with masters degree level training contribute an enormous amount to the administration and management of research and disease control programs, but this paper assumes that their activities are in general outside the sphere of policy-making and planning.

There is general agreement within academic and scientific circles that an existing national shortage of epidemiologists and biostatisticians will worsen in the near future. Demands for their services are bound to increase during the next few years, and these increased demands will coincide with reduced numbers of graduates because present cutbacks in training have imposed constraints that will carry over for three to five years or longer. There is also an impression of general consensus that fundamental reasons for existing shortages go far beyond recent changes in federal funding policies. In 1959, long before wide-scale application of epidemiology and health statistics to planning and management of personal health services, the National Institute of General Medical Sciences Advisory Committee on Epidemiology and Biometry estimated a needed annual output of 75 graduates with masters or doctoral degrees in one or the other of the two disciplines (1). Its program was designed to support the training of this number of scientists. It was not possible, however, to maintain trainee enrollment to meet the scheduled output, and until very recently the decline in reported dollar expenditures over time was as much a consequence as a cause of decreasing annual numbers of graduates.

Table 6–1 below shows the trend in the numbers of institutional training grants in epidemiology from 1958 to 1978.

Table 6–1. Institutional Training Grants in Epidemiology—1958–78

School Year	1958–59	1961–62	1964–65	1967–68	1970–71	1974–75	1977–78
Number of Grants	11	19	20	10	8	5	0

In an effort to encourage recruitment of trainees into the discipline of epidemiology the Institute sponsored new centers of education in veterinary, medical, and dental schools and introduced summer fellowship programs for medical students. In spite of the enthusiasm of the directors and students of some of these programs, their overall impact on recruiting has been negligible. They did, however, act as conceptual forerunners of the Clinical Scholars program to broaden the base of education and hopefully the attitudes and interests of future clinical specialists.

It is important to note that the failure to fill available training slots in epidemiology described above did not apply to biostatistics. Consequently, the recent federal decision to discontinue training support had a relatively greater impact on biometry. The number of institutional grants in biometry will be cut by two-thirds (four instead of twelve) between 1974–75 (2) and 1977–78. The converse is also true. Reinstatement of funds and programs will have a much more rapid and predictable impact on biostatistical than on epidemiological manpower reserves.

During the last five years schools of medicine slowly began to recognize national interest in personal health service delivery programs designed to meet community needs. That recognition is slowly growing into acceptance of the inevitable introduction of management and evaluation techniques into health care delivery organizations and systems. Some of their departments of preventive medicine became almost evan-

gelistic about the development of residency training programs designed
to bring epidemiological and management strategies and skills into the
clinical training arena. This burgeoning interest of medical schools is reflected in the current distribution of formal general preventive medicine residency training programs which include epidemiology (Table
6–2) (3).

**Table 6–2. Residency Training Programs Which Include Epidemiology—
1975**

Institution	Number of Programs
Medical Schools	8
Public Health Schools	6
Combined Programs	3
Federal Programs	3
Total	20

Twenty of the twenty-six active general preventive medicine residency-
training programs in this country in 1975 claim to emphasize epidemiology and its application. Eight are in schools of medicine, three are
jointly sponsored by schools of medicine and public health, six are in
schools of public health per se, and three are in federal agencies (Center
for Disease Control, Walter Reed Army Medical Center, and Brooks Air
Force Base). All twenty program directors were interviewed by tele-
phone in January 1975. The directors in the eleven medical schools
shared an opinion that overall recruitment is a greater limitation than
money—a relatively dramatic consensus when Public Health Service
Training funds are virtually nonexistent. Six of the eight independent
medical school programs find it virtually impossible to recruit graduating
physicians into their residency slots. The other two have numerous applicants, but the majority do not meet their departmental admission criteria. The three jointly sponsored programs have few medically qualified
applicants, and directors of programs in schools of public health as a
group find it even harder to attract medical graduates than do directors
of programs in schools of medicine. The numbers of available places
for trainees and the numbers of current trainees in these twenty programs are summarized in Table 6–3.

Table 6-3. Residency Training Programs—1975

Institution	Number of Places	Number of Trainees	Projected Number of Practicing Epidemiologists*
Medical Schools	22	10	5
Public Health Schools	not stated	10	10
Combined Programs	6	5	5
Federal Programs	26	17	7
Total	54	42	27

* Estimate by program directors.

Even when training slots are filled many trainees do not specialize in epidemiology. There are two explanations for this phenomenon. Several programs teach limited amounts of epidemiology within the context of specific training for such careers as industrial or aerospace medicine. In others the loss of earmarked training support has led to increased use of patient care and research monies to support residents. The work they do to justify their support turns their career development toward the use of epidemiology within clinical practice or medical administration, and away from epidemiology as an investigative science. A few additional trainees were identified in the medical school, federal, and combined programs. They are summarized in Table 6-4.

Table 6-4. Other Trainees—1975

Institution	M.D.	Non-M.D.
Medical Schools	3	12
Combined Programs	1	–
Federal Programs	7	–
Total Epidemiologists	11	12

The numbers are insignificant in light of currently projected needs. All schools of public health in the United States were surveyed by Winkelstein in February 1975 (4). Their 1975 outputs of graduates with doctoral degrees in epidemiology will be fourteen physicians and twenty-one nonphysicians (Table 6–5).

Table 6–5. Doctoral Candidates—1975*

	M.D.	Other
Public Health Schools	14	21

* Preliminary figures.

Both the medical and public health school surveys asked for estimates of maximum epidemiologist training capacity if all necessary faculty and student support was made available. The estimates given by the schools are summarized in Table 6–6.

Table 6–6. Maximum Training Capacity—1975

Institution	Residents	Doctoral Candidates
Medical Schools	38	–
Public Health Schools	18	56*
Combined Programs	20	–
Federal Programs	64	–
Total	140	56

* Estimated on the basis of present Doctoral/Masters candidate ratio.

Berg surveyed medical school faculties in 1971 and reported a deficit of 200 epidemiologists (1). He estimated a need for 135 to 195 graduates in epidemiology in each of the next nine years and 60 to 120 in each subsequent year to bring the medical schools to capacity and maintain them at the working level of four epidemiologists per school. The 1975 figures described above suggest that our total national resources could do no more than maintain the early 1970 level of medical school staffing, a level deemed appropriate before student bodies increased to their maximum size and before Professional Standards Review Organizations (PSRO's) and other types of evaluation became daily requirements in clinical services. The lack of interest of United States medical school graduates in epidemiology described by training program directors is further documented in Levit's description of the specialty choice of graduating 1960 and 1964 medical school cohorts (5). Nine of 640 (1960) and ten of 673 (1964) graduates designated preventive medicine as their specialty. Given that approximately one in ten general preventive medicine specialists is an epidemiologist, one in each of these medical school cohorts became an epidemiologist. There are a number of very obvious reasons for our national failure to recruit and develop an appropriate complement of physician epidemiologists. Our training centers have been conceptually, physically and professionally isolated from medical students. The medical students have, therefore, been left without role models to alert them to the specialty as a career opportunity. Within the medical profession epidemiology, particularly as applied to clinical practice, is a relatively new specialty. A majority of established clinical specialists and practitioners were educated before it was widely introduced into medical school curricula. Low visibility, coupled with lack of understanding of its applications, virtually insures its absence in clinical conferences and research. In the field of infectious diseases and drug trials, chronic overall shortages have limited opportunities for other physicians to work with epidemiologists on a day-to-day basis. As a consequence medical schools have been slow to require competent education in the discipline. In 1974 only 75 per cent of the United States medical schools required at least one course in epidemiology (6). A majority of these courses simply provided descriptive material which gives little insight into the problem definition and solving capabilities of the discipline and the impact it can, and should, have on medical decisions and the practice of medicine. Most general and specialized training in epidemiology is provided in nonclinical settings. This separation of training and its research basis from clinical activities has endowed epidemiologists with basic science salaries and relatively low prestige within the medical centers where students make their career selections. The postdoctoral trainee in a school of public health gets a much lower stipend than a clinical resident or postdoctoral fellow. Differences in earning capacity continue during career development. These disparities between the incomes of epidemiologists and other medical specialists are increasing as more and more medical centers provide their clinical faculties with opportunities to earn additional income from private practice to compensate for institutional inability to increase full-time salaries in line with inflationary costs of living.

Although there is agreement about shortages and reasons for shortages, there is a range of opinion about the dimensions of the shortage and the necessary proportions of physician versus nonphysician epidemiologists in the future. Points of argument are often more emotional than rational because any national decisions to promote physician epidemiologists will have a dramatic impact on schools of public health. They will either have to reduce their masters level training responsibilities and develop intimate relationships with their medical school counterparts or concentrate on the education of masses of middle-level public health practitioners and a limited output of nonphysician epidemiologists who will assume public health practice responsibilities and carry out some epidemiological research. The amount of etiologic research that can be undertaken by nonphysicians is determined by the extent to which an understanding of the natural history and pathophysiological mechanisms of disease is a requirement for the development of rational etiological hypotheses. As technology in the basic biomedical sciences has improved, diagnosis has moved closer to the cellular than the organ system level. Consequently, prospects for detection of disease susceptibles and for prevention of disease have been dramatically increased. However, investigative questions will have to be phrased in the context and terms of modern cell biology to capitalize on and exploit this new knowledge. These advances point in many ways to an increasing rather than decreasing need for physician versus nonphysician epidemiologists to engage in "classical" studies of cause and control of disease.

Some new applications of epidemiological strategies will be needed to support our national 1976–80 priority goals. These new applications are also likely to demand proportionately more physician epidemiologists. Prevention is the first priority mentioned in the Forward Plan (7). Dr. Lewis Thomas's 1972 statement that prevention only comes from genuine understanding of the disease mechanism (8) and Dr. Theodore Cooper's very recent statement that measures of prevention within our modern culture must be clearly justified on the basis of efficacy (9) suggest that training in both medicine and epidemiology are prerequisites for decisions about advances in this area. Knowledge of the distribution and consequences of disease is a fundamental cornerstone of any population-based health insurance program. Preparation for national health insurance is another quoted national priority. Although there is room for differences of opinion about the best measures to use to assess needs of populations for health services, there can be no disagreement that scientists trained to measure, classify, and monitor disease in populations have critical roles to play in the collection of evidence to establish priorities in the allocation of resources for the best community impact.

A great deal of experimental epidemiological research is necessary to develop useful measures of the efficacy of intervention at different stages in the natural history of major diseases. These measures are the only valid basis for assessment of the quality of intervention, another national priority. In spite of rapid technological developments in computer and information sciences there has been little constructive application to the health industry. The conceptualization, planning, and implementation of information systems to provide administrators and policy-makers with information to describe the progress of the public's health during the next several decades is a long overdue priority. Its rapid implementation has major short- and long-term implications for the supply of health statisticians. There is an obvious need for the engagement of epidemiologists and biostatisticians in development of new knowledge about environmental hazards and the natural history of disease processes. These two areas of the Forward Plan emphasis fall into the purview of classical epidemiological research. Proposals for support of this latter type of research are submitted to the National Institutes of Health and reviewed by the Epidemiology and Disease Control Study Section. This Study Section and the program staff of the Institutes have shared a growing concern, both about the relative shortage of proposals submitted for support of research into the causes of such important diseases as cancer and chronic lung disease, and about the low proportion of submitted proposals that warrant approval. A detailed study of research proposals reviewed by the Epidemiology and Disease Control Study Section during the years 1969 and 1970 pinpointed some major reasons for their poor technical quality. Only 26 per cent of reviewed grants were submitted by fully qualified investigators (for this analysis a qualified investigator had doctoral or postdoctoral training in epidemiology, biostatistics, or applied sociology). An additional 21 per cent of the 132 proposals reviewed were submitted by investigators with minimal training in one or another of the three disciplines. In other words, only one in four proposals for funds to carry out epidemiological research was prepared by a qualified epidemiologist or biostatistician, and more than half were prepared by applicants with absolutely no training in either discipltne. The members of the Study Section learned through site visits and anecdotal information that the faculties and staffs of many medical institutions have no access whatsoever to competent epidemiological and/or biostatistical collaboration or even consultation. Even worse, large numbers of applicants failed to realize the need for such collaboration and/or consultation (Table 6–7).

Several other important investigative questions listed in the Forward Plan fall into the domain of health services research. An analysis of a sample of research proposals reviewed by the Health Services Research Study Section during 1972–75 showed an almost insignificant involvement of epidemiologists and biostatisticians. Table 6–8 shows that one

Table 6–7. Epidemiology and Disease Control Research Proposals Reviewed at Seven Study Section Meetings in 1969–70

	Number of Proposals	Per Cent
Total Proposals	132	100
Proposals with Qualified Investigator(s)*	33	26
Proposals with Investigators Having Minimal Disciplinary Training	28	21
Other	71	53

* For this analysis, a "qualified" investigator had doctoral or postdoctoral training in epidemiology, biostatistics, or applied sociology.

or the other discipline was included in 14 per cent of the proposals and that their low participation rates were consistent over these three years.

The virtual absence of epidemiologists and biostatisticians from the growing field of health services research in this country is probably a consequence both of short supply and of physical separation from medical centers and ongoing health care delivery programs.

These opportunities to assess from two perspectives the volume and quality of classical epidemiological research interests and the extent of expressed interest of epidemiologists and biostatisticians in the application of epidemiological strategies within the field of health services

Table 6–8. Health Services Research Proposals—1972–75

	Number	Per Cent
Total Proposals	177	100.0
Proposals with an Epidemiologist*	15	8.5
Proposals with a Biostatistician*	18	10.0
Proposals with either an Epidemiologist or a Biostatistician	25	14.0
Other	152	86.0

* These are not exclusive groups.

Table 6–9. Ratio of U.S./Foreign Medical Graduates by Age Among Full-Time Public Health School Epidemiology Faculty—1974–75

Age (years)	Ratio U.S./Foreign Medical Graduates
30–39	3 : 1
40–49	4 : 1
50 and over	3 : 1

research provide both additional evidence of an acute shortage of well-trained scientists and additional reasons to question the wisdom of training them outside centers which have ongoing clinical activities. Since the 1950's epidemiology has attracted high proportions of graduates of foreign medical schools. If, as is very likely, steps are taken to reduce career opportunities for foreign medical graduates in the United States, there will have to be a relatively greater increase in the recruitment of United States graduates than currently projected.

An analysis of the full-time faculties of departments of epidemiology in all the United States schools of public health showed a consistent ratio of 1 foreign to 3–4 United States medical graduates (Table 6–9). In addition, these physician-epidemiologists were old compared with all United States physicians (Table 6–10).

Their greater age is partly explained by long years of training for those who train in a clinical specialty before epidemiology, but it may in part indicate a need to consider stepped-up short-term recruitment to maintain current faculty levels over the next twenty years.

The majority of biostatisticians are educated in schools of public health. Even though the absolute number of full-time faculty in departments of biostatistics in schools of public health has increased, the rate

Table 6–10. Cumulative Per Cent Distribution of Ages of all Physicians in the United States and Physician-Epidemiologists in the United States Schools of Public Health—1974–75

Age (years)	Physicians (%)	Physician-Epidemiologists (%)
Less than 40	39	23
Less than 50	63	52

of increase has lagged far behind the rate of increase of the student body. The first and most frightening effect of understaffing is on doctoral level programs which require major allocations of faculty time. The following figures are estimates for departments of biostatistics in all United States schools of public health except Puerto Rico (Table 6–11).

Table 6–11. Departments of Biostatistics in the United States

Year	Full-Time Faculty	Students All	Doctoral	Faculty/Student Ratio All	Doctoral
1968–69	82	55	7	1.5	11.7
1969–70	97	72	25	1.3	3.9
1974–75	138	158	41	0.9	3.4

Disparities between industrial and academic biostatistical salaries have been increasing rapidly while conditions of academic life, particularly for good doctoral education, have been deteriorating. The effect of these two forces is a 1974–75 vacancy rate of 10 per cent among budgeted biostatistical faculty positions in United States schools of public health (4). The figures in Table 6–12 give estimates of the capacity of United States schools of public health to educate doctoral-level biostatisticians. The 1974 estimate of the pool of applicants suggests that if existing programs were boosted to capacity they could accept all available candidates. To do so would require reconsideration both of faculty salaries compared to industrial salaries and a reduction in the teaching time allocated to nondoctoral students.

However, the pool of applicants falls far short of estimated overall needs for graduates in biostatistics and additional attention must be given both to recruitment and to training program expansion. The schools of public health can easily expand their doctoral programs if they are willing to make marked reductions in numbers of masters-level

Table 6–12. Capacity to Educate Doctoral Candidates in Departments of Biostatistics with the Pool of Applicants—1974–75

Capacity*	Pool of Applicants
164	134

* Estimated on present Masters/Doctoral candidate ratios.

students. If they do, who will train the operating, technical, and middle management biostatisticians? They are similarly in short supply and likely to become more scarce. The venues of technical and practical training versus more didactic education become a matter of national policy. The same decision has to be made for biostatistics and epidemiology: will schools of public health become technical schools and other programs educate the academicians, or will technical schools be used to relieve the schools of public health of some of their burden in this respect and allow them to expand their doctoral enrollment?

Whether we accept the estimates developed by Kerr White (10) or those published by the University of North Carolina in 1973 (11), there is no doubt that our present training resources are inadequate both in capacity and resources, and that they fail to provide attractive education and career opportunities.

We are beginning to see limited efforts to introduce training within categorical programs, an approach which is more in line with residency training in other specialties. The National Center for Health Services Research has had experience with approximately 103 trainees. There is some tentative evidence that this approach at least succeeds in keeping the graduates in academic and administrative careers (12). The fellowship training program of the National Cancer Institute is virtually too small to assess any impact (13). But its new training programs within clinical cancer centers can provide unique opportunities to evaluate their potential to recruit into clinical settings. If these settings do attract trainees, our slowly developing program of regionalized clinical research and demonstration centers may provide the potential for innovative and competitive training programs. Whether or not medical centers of one kind or another prove to be the best venues for training programs, the questions of peer status, prestige, and income will have to be answered before epidemiology can compete on equal terms for our medical school graduates.

References

1. National Institute of General Medical Sciences, Epidemiology and Biometry Training Committee, "Manpower Needs for Epidemiologists" (July 1971). Unpublished Report.

2. M. Carlson, Personal Communication (January 1975).

3. American Medical Association Directory of Approved Internships and Residencies 1973–74 (Chicago, Ill.: A.M.A., 1974), and R. Tracy, Personal Communication (January 1975).

4. W. Winkelstein, Personal Communication (February 1975).

5. E. J. Levit, M. Sabshin, and C. B. Mueller, "Trends in Graduate Medical Education and Specialty Certification. A Tracking Study of United States Medical School Graduates," *New England Journal of Medicine* 290 (1974), 545–49.

6. W. H. Barker, "ATPM Survey," *ATPM Newsletter* 21, No. 1 (1974), 10–14.

7. United States Department of Health, Education and Welfare, Office of the Assistant Secretary for Health, *Forward Plan for Health, FY 1976–80* (Washington, D.C.: GPO, 1974).

8. L. Thomas, "Aspects of Biomedical Science Policy," Occasional Paper, National Academy of Sciences, Institute of Medicine (Washington, D.C., 1972). Processed.

9. T. Cooper, Deputy Assistant Secretary for Health, Department of Health, Education, and Welfare, Anglo-American Conference on Priorities in Medicine, Planning Committee Meeting (Bethesda, Md.: Fogarty International Center, Feb. 5, 1975). Processed.

10. K. L. White, "Opportunities and Needs for Epidemiology and Health Statistics in the United States," in *Epidemiology as a Fundamental Science: Its Uses in Health Services Planning, Administration, and Evaluation*, eds. K. L. White and M. M. Henderson (New York: Oxford Univ. Press, 1976) pp. 66–77.

11. Task Force on Professional Health Manpower, *Professional Health Manpower for Community Health Programs*, Univ. of North Carolina School of Public Health, Dept. of Health Administration (Chapel Hill: Univ. of North Carolina, 1973).

12. G. Rosenthal, Personal Communication (February 1975).

13. H. Densen, Personal Communication (February 1975).

Discussion

Opening Remarks: Edward A. Mortimer, M.D.

The decrease in funding for training in epidemiology and biometry pre-sents an incredible paradox in that, at a time when the Federal Govern-ment displays maximum and commendable concern about the goals of medical care, it is at the same time indiscriminately cutting back on the training of the very group of professionals who can contribute most to reducing its costs, the epidemiologists and biometrists. From my standpoint as a clinician I refer not only to such enterprises as the evalu-ation of community programs and their cost-benefit ratios, but also to the pragmatic value of the epidemiological approach to the direct care of patients. To me one of the critical deficits in the United States today is that of the failure of our schools of medicine to imbue their stu-dents with epidemiological concepts and methods. Some basic epidemi-ological knowledge on the part of our physicians could, I believe, cut the costs of medical care by one-third. One example may clarify my reasoning: tonsillectomy and adenoidectomy. In Albuquerque, New

Mexico, with a population of one-third million, one out of three children reaches adulthood without his tonsils. The annual cost of "therapy" is one million dollars. The value of this legalized, socially acceptable form of child abuse is so limited that it can no longer be justified for more than one or two per cent of children. The very little epidemiological knowledge needed to understand this is not acquired by physicians in training. Further, as noted by Geiger (New York Times, March 2, 1975), one of our major health service problems is that the supplier of medical care, the physician, is also the individual who creates the demand by determining who goes to the hospital, what tests to perform, and what therapy to administer. This supplier must learn and use epidemiology.

The lack of qualified applicants for training in epidemiology perhaps stems from the fact that medical students have little or no exposure to epidemiology in medical school and house officer training. Medical schools are dominated by departments focused on the care and study of individual patients whose faculties are unaware of the rudiments of epidemiology.

Dr. Henderson's data are correct about the number of grant applications lacking epidemiological and biostatistical components. However, once again it depends on which part of the elephant one palpates. Some of the applications with excellent epidemiological and biostatistical design and support were grossly defective in core medical support. When I completed my term on the Epidemiology and Disease Control Study Section, a colleague and I wrote a grant application that we thought would be enthusiastically cheered by the Study Section for its epidemiological planning. Unfortunately it went to the Bacteriology Study Section rather than to the Epidemiology and Disease Control Study Section, and here it was quite poorly received because that Study Section could not identify an investigator whom they considered to exhibit proper bacteriological qualifications.

I think the message here of a definite need for greater interrelationships with other disciplines is clear; as a gross generalization teachers of medicine do not know epidemiology, and epidemiologists do not know medicine.

Summary of General Discussion

1. *Clinical scholars.*
With reference to clinical scholars, the problem is to get them to achieve competence both clinically and as scholars. In the program at The Johns Hopkins University there have been essentially two groups:

those who were in fact scholars and able to learn to distinguish the worthwhile from the useless; in the second group there have been a number of activists who had great difficulty in separating science from activism. Both are required to accomplish change. It is difficult to see how clinical scholars can really be scholars if they develop in an environment where there is very little in the way of skepticism, critical judgment or objective approaches to questions of care, not to mention knowledge of the methods and concepts of investigation. These barriers need crossing. There may come a day when every clinical department has two or three epidemiologically oriented members with an intellectual concern with population medicine at one end of the medical science spectrum that is equal to the current intellectual concerns at the opposite end of the spectrum that focus on molecular events.

It seems rather strange that the relationship of the quantitative sciences to clinical knowledge has not developed in a manner similar to the development of the biological sciences in relation to clinical medicine. The precedent is there, and the opportunities exist, yet it is commonplace, as has been implied, for professors of medicine and surgery to go on teaching truisms that are not truisms at all, such as the abuse of tonsillectomy mentioned by Dr. Mortimer.

Payment methods have drastically distorted the system in the United States. As long as there is so much gain connected with surgery, for example, and so little connected with the type of professional and scientific input being discussed here, distortion is bound to continue. The institutional arrangements and systems of incentives and rewards must change in a very basic way in this area.

2. *Comments on the difficulty of attracting qualified people to epidemiology.*

There appears to be quite a lot of interest in quantitative medicine among medical students provided they are able to see an outlet for these interests somewhere in the future. However, they seem to find it extremely difficult to know where they can, in fact, function if they choose career training in this direction. The reward system has a great deal to do with this, and if one looks at what has happened to the public health system in the United States in many areas, it becomes easy to understand why they do not see a very clear role to play. It would seem that public health departments have been more or less written off as laws are passed to substitute for them in one way or another through Regional Medical Programs or Comprehensive Health Planning Agencies, all of which seem to have a rather peripheral relationship to the organized health care system. Until the career epidemiologist has a place in which to function, it will be extremely difficult to find many highly qualified people who will assess the future career situation as a good opportunity.

It was noted as exceptional, however, that while the Department of Health Care Organization of The Johns Hopkins School of Hygiene and Public Health accepted only eight or nine graduate students in 1975, about 160 inquiries and 50 or 60 firm applications were received, indicating the existence of a huge pool of candidates, perhaps not all properly qualified, but interested.

Further increasing the general difficulty of recruiting qualified people is the perceived lack of attractiveness associated with many of the training programs offered. In many cases people looking for suitable training programs are discouraged by the fact that many are by no means as rigorous or as relevant as the candidates think they need to be in order to prepare them to work in the health care system of the future. Perhaps the training programs should be strengthened and thereby increase the attractiveness of epidemiology.

3. *Issues and questions.*

The issue of whether or not the epidemiologist wants to "sell" epidemiology must be kept to the fore, and the problem must be defined.

Recruitment is an issue that relates to the profile of the person being trained and to the function that person is going to fill. The problems of financing and salary levels follow and do not precede recruitment, because if the types of people needed cannot be attracted by defining the functions, then, in turn, they cannot be trained.

Dr. Anderson and Dr. Knox have said that epidemiology is changing. It may be changing in their worlds, but is it changing in the United States?

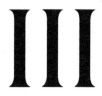

III

ADMINISTRATIVE
APPLICATIONS
OF EPIDEMIOLOGY
AND HEALTH STATISTICS,
AND THE TRAINING
OF ADMINISTRATORS

7

ROY M. ACHESON, M.D.

EPIDEMIOLOGY:
THE TRAINING OF
COMMUNITY PHYSICIANS
IN GREAT BRITAIN

Background

The present approach to the graduate and postgraduate teaching of epidemiology in Britain stems from the same slow changes in social and professional outlook that led to the reorganization of the National Health Service (NHS) in April 1974. Scotland was ahead of the rest of Great Britain, both in terms of legislation for reorganization and in the training program which preceded it (1, 2). In England, with which, in the interests of brevity, this paper must be chiefly concerned, one of the most important facets of the new NHS legislation has been the decentralization of responsibility for budgeting and planning for the day-to-day running of the service. The basic administrative unit in the service is the district, the national norm for which is a population of 250,000, and a general hospital which provides the most important of the specialist clinical services. In practice, for historical, geographical, and demographic reasons many districts deviate from this norm. There are between one and six districts in an area, and areas are grouped into fourteen regions. Although the formulation of policy is the responsibility of Area Authorities, who are appointed bodies of lay people each with a lay chairman, the administration of the health service in each district is in the hands of a peer group of six people, an administrator, finance officer, nurse, two clinical doctors, and the district community physician, who must work by consensus. Thus, the daily planning and management of the service is in the hands of groups of professionals who are in a position to intimately match health needs to resources at the local level. Probably a quarter-century has passed since it was foreseen that epidemiology would become a key instrument in the effective planning of health services. Now it is the task of the community physicians in each of some 200 health districts to learn to use this instrument for this purpose. Unlike the United States, where the chief emphasis of graduate instruction is on the use of epidemiology in etiological research and disease control, the tendency in England today is to pay increasing attention to its use in the planning and evaluation of health services.

Reorganization of Medical Education

During the years when the seeds of change which preceded the reorganization of the health service were being sown, a Royal Commission was convened, which recommended that extensive modifications should be made in medical education (3). At the graduate and postgraduate levels some of these did little more than bring Great Britain into line with procedures which for many years have been commonplace in the United States; others were more far-reaching. Community medicine was defined, and it was recommended that a central body should be formed with a responsibility for setting standards in, and overseeing the quality of, postgraduate education and training in this field throughout Great Britain and Northern Ireland. It also recommended that, in line with clinical specialties, this body should operate through a regional organization. As a consequence of these recommendations and of extensive negotiations between the interested professional organizations, in 1972 the Royal Colleges of Physicians of London, Edinburgh, and Glasgow established a Faculty of Community Medicine as the central body that the commission considered necessary. It is important to realize that the British concept of community medicine differs fundamentally from that of the United States. The faculty's definition, which incorporates minor modifications of the Royal Commission's, is as follows:

> Community medicine is that branch of medicine which deals with populations or groups rather than individual patients. In the context of a national system of medical care, it therefore comprises those doctors who try to measure accurately the needs of the population both sick and well.

It requires to bring to the study special knowledge of the principles of epidemiology, of the organization and evaluation of medical care systems, of the medical aspects of the administration of health services and of the techniques of health education and rehabilitation which are comprised within the field of social and preventive medicine.

Community medicine thus brings together within one discipline those who are presently engaged in the practice of public health, in the administration of the health services, whether in hospital, local authority, or central government, in relevant research, and those responsible for undergraduate and postgraduate education in the university departments of social medicine.

Educational Policy of the Faculty of Community Medicine

The faculty has introduced a membership examination (MFCM) which has qualities in common with the membership examinations of the parent Colleges of Physicians. Moreover, just as membership in the Royal Colleges of Physicians is a parallel qualification to Board Certification in Internal Medicine in the United States, so membership in the Faculty of Community Medicine is now nationally accepted in Britain as indicative of completed early specialist training in that field. In addition, it has already attracted a good deal of interest overseas.

The examination is in two parts. The present curriculum for the first part has been published by the faculty and is described in detail elsewhere by Warren and Acheson (4). Candidates must answer a written examination on epidemiology and statistics (which are accepted as being the basic sciences of community medicine), on social sciences as they relate to community medicine, and on the principles of administration and management. The second part, usually completed at least a year after the first, is taken by submitting a written report on a research investigation in which the candidate must demonstrate his ability to apply the scientific skills upon which he was examined in Part I to a problem in community medicine and by undergoing an oral examination on his report. Recent publications (5–9) give, in some detail, views on the scientific content of community medicine with emphasis on the contribution of epidemiology. This work must be undertaken with the advice of a tutor who has been approved by the faculty; the proposed title and research outline must also be approved in advance.

Experience with both parts of the examination is still limited, but it is probably true to say that the standard required in Part II is broadly equivalent to that required in North American schools of public health for the doctoral degree in public health (Dr.P.H. or D.Sc.). It is certainly much higher than the standard formerly required in British medical schools for the diploma in public health. The methods used for training candidates for this examination are still in the developmental stage. Candidates for Part I need not do any formal course work and are at liberty to attempt it on the basis of private study if they so choose. Clearly, however, most candidates prefer to have an opportunity to study in groups under direction, and it is important that the most effective possible use is made of the limited academic resources in the country. In Britain, as in the United States, there are still some medical schools which are totally lacking in effective undergraduate medical education in epidemiology and public health, though the proportion of these in Britain is smaller than that in the United States. In Great Britain, however, four medical schools (two of which are in Scotland) offer graduate programs in community medicine which lead to university qualifications and which through 1977 will carry exemption from Part I of the MFCM because the faculty was satisfied that the examination set in each school covers the same ground as is stipulated in the MFCM curriculum. The one graduate school of public health in the country, the London School of Hygiene and Tropical Medicine, has since 1969 been offering a two-year master's course which prepares candidates for a career in community medicine, and those who successfully complete this course before 1977 are also exempt. After 1977 the faculty will decide whether to continue to offer exemption to graduates of these or any other schools, or whether it will require all candidates for the MFCM to take the faculty's own examination. However, no exemptions are granted from the second part; although candidates may, if they choose, submit the same material as has been submitted for university qualifications.

It had been foreseen by a special government working party on medical administration, the Hunter Committee (10), that it would be unlikely that the training capacity of individual schools would be sufficient to meet the immediate needs of the National Health Service for trained community physicians, let alone the needs for teachers; this has proved to be the case. Other medical schools throughout the country have therefore arranged themselves in three groups or consortia, one in the midlands and southwest, one in London and the southeast, and one in the north, to provide additional training programs. Trainees are appointed to residencies in community medicine attached to an area or region in the part of the country concerned and receive a salary from the National Health Service. It takes one-and-a-half to two years to complete the course work for Part I of the MFCM, and each of the collaborating universities in the consortium contributes by teaching that part of the curriculum in which it has special expertise. Time between courses is devoted to in-service training. Training by the consortia is entirely directed toward the MFCM examination; at the moment there is no way for trainees under this scheme to obtain a university degree. One great advantage of the scheme is that it enables small academic departments of community medicine (and most such departments are small) to participate in graduate education without accepting the huge, if not impossible, task of carrying the responsibility for running a full-time course. There are disadvantages, however. Considerable overlaps exist in the resources of the collaborating schools and universities. In general, it is easier to promote courses in epidemiology than in health economics or medical sociology, although university departments outside medical schools are contributing to the teaching of these subjects. The scheme is still at an experimental and developmental stage; one consortium recruited its first trainees in the fall of 1973, the second in the fall of 1974, and the third did not start work until the fall of 1975. It will, therefore, be some time before trainees complete their work and a proper evaluation can be made of the programs. It is hoped that in the future most trainees will enter the field after two or three years of clinical experience in hospital or general practice, or even better, both. At the moment some recruits have done clinical work for much longer.

Continuing Education and Postgraduate Training

In 1968 when the Royal Commission published its report (3), continuing education in medicine in general compared poorly in Great Britain with that in the United States, but both countries had in common an almost total absence of organized continuing education in public health or in social or community medicine. As soon as it was known that the commission had laid special emphasis on the need to develop this aspect of education in Great Britain, several schools began to develop plans. Among them was the London School of Hygiene and Tropical Medicine which, stimulated by Dr. J. N. Morris, put forward proposals to the Department of Health and Social Security for the development of a center whose specific full-time responsibility was to offer postgraduate training and continuing education in community medicine. The need for such a program was endorsed by the report of the Hunter Committee (10). The center came into being with the appointment of a director and an administrator in July 1972 and as of the present has given about thirty courses varying in length from five weeks to one day. In addition, it has produced publications on a limited basis, some of which have drawn upon special advanced seminars given in the center; it has also initiated a small research program.

The Work of the London Centre for Extension Training In Community Medicine

Preparing for Reorganization. All the center's activities have been strongly influenced by the national convulsions accompanying the reorganization of the health service. When the center opened, the Department of Health and Social Security had, with the help of the Universities of Birmingham, Manchester, and the National University of Wales, already embarked upon a crash program to retrain senior public health physicians and medically qualified administrators from the hospital service, to prepare them for the tasks they would face when the Health Act became law. High among the skills they were to master was the ability to apply epidemiology to the planning and evaluation of health services. For many this was a new challenge; all the public health physicians were experienced in the use of epidemiology in infectious disease control, and the less senior of them had also received instruction in chronic disease epidemiology. The hospital service physicians had had little reason to use epidemiology. Most of the preparatory courses in the program lasted only four weeks during which time many topics other than epidemiology were covered, including management techniques, planning methods, health economics, and the basis of reorganization itself.

Present program. The preparatory phase ended at the beginning of April 1974 when the service was reorganized and theory became practice. That spring and summer the center started an ongoing program which involves the detailed study of how practice differs from theory. During the preparatory phase, training was based on the interpretation of reports of committees and working parties and on government circulars. Extensive reorganization must bring with it new appointments and new roles. The tasks each of the community physicians and specialists in community medicine were expected to perform were outlined by the Department of Health and Social Security in a series of "job profiles." But as soon as people began to do these tasks the views of government officers about what *should* happen immediately assumed an importance which was no greater than what actually *was* happening. Thus if the center's teaching is to retain credibility it is critical that its staff should remain closely in touch with developments, and it does this partly by running a series of carefully planned but loosely structured seminars, in which community physicians with a wide range of responsibilities have the opportunity to discuss their tasks and responsibilities. The center is also carrying out questionnaire surveys, on a national basis, of community physicians as well as of some of the groups constituting the new service. The necessity for these surveys lies in the fact that the present demand is for short vocational courses; and it is possible that there is a demand for longer courses for district community physicians, medical specialists in social services, medical information officers, and so forth. It is hoped that these continuing studies will also have long-term value in guiding the work of the center.

Keeping up to date. The scientific basis of community medicine has been evolving from the needs of a previous, vastly different form of the National Health Service and a different climate of medical and academic thinking. The present curriculum is therefore only a step toward the future. It will indeed be surprising if practitioners of the various subspecialties of community medicine do not feel a need to master various skills and disciplines which are not immediately obvious. Moreover science itself will not stand still. Doubtless the faculty will from time to time take cognizance of this by changing the basic syllabus for the MFCM. Such changes obviously can be of no direct benefit to those who already have the MFCM and hold senior posts in the Service. The center considers it to be one of its responsibilities to keep abreast of developments in related fields so that it can offer both refresher courses in those sciences basic to community medicine with which community physicians are already familiar as well as others in appropriate disciplines which are new to them.

Future plans. The jargon of the teaching faculty of the center itself is to refer to the vocational courses described above as "course *for*" and to the discipline-specific courses just described as "courses *on*." A move toward the presentation of "courses on" is to be made during the forthcoming year (1975–76), and preparations are already being made for a course on the behavioral and social sciences as they relate to community medicine and another on epidemiology and statistics. It should follow from these facts that the content of both these courses will almost certainly differ considerably from courses with similar titles which have been given elsewhere.

Teaching methods. The age of the student is a most important determinant of appropriate methods for teaching. It is well known that mature adults learn more slowly than those in early adult life. On the other hand, they have acquired a great deal of experience and knowledge which neither their classmates nor their teachers may have. For these two reasons the center adopted the policy of reducing formal didactic presentations to a minimum and making maximum use of small group work. Not only has this allowed students to work at their own speed by teaching each other and the faculty of the center, but it has also allowed the careful and informed consideration of a wide variety of problems to which there is not, and in some instances may never be, an official answer. A great difficulty about this approach is that it is practically impossible to evaluate objectively what has been achieved. Students will finish courses with a wide variety of new facts, and perhaps attitudes, which frequently they did not expect to acquire, and more often they do not even realize they have acquired.

Epidemiology in Community Medicine

It was stated at the outset that one of the principal users of the epidemiological approach in the reorganized National Health Service will be the district community physician (DCP) although his colleagues at region and area level will use it too. At present and for the foreseeable future, the DCP's supporting staff will be limited to a very few untrained office workers. For this reason alone, there is no question of his embarking on special surveys of any kind, either for the identification of need or for evaluation. He must rely on readily available information. New methods are being developed for providing this information, including a relatively simple but comprehensive computerized set of data relating to all hospital inpatients the analysis of which is organized on a regional basis (11, 12); this system is working quite well in some parts of the country but is having serious teething troubles elsewhere. The DCP must learn the enormous potential of this system, the most important part of which is known as hospital activity analysis (12). He must learn not only to consider morbid phenomena in terms of the human population, but also to consider them in relation to the population of available beds, to available manpower, and to other resources. Bed occupancy rate and "throughput" per bed per year (i.e., numbers of patients cared for per available bed) are after all identical mathematical concepts to prevalence and incidence and both have the same relationship to time. Admittedly it is easier to plan methods of changing the events which underlie the statistics when beds are the denominator than it is to change the rates of disease in the population. Similarly he must be prepared to be flexible in his manner of including in his calculations the medical manpower force and inanimate resources such as hospitals and clinics. The Office of Population Censuses and Surveys provides annual estimates of local populations which are of considerable value to health planning in their own right. The accuracy of these will be enhanced by the fact that it is proposed to carry out national censuses at five- rather than ten-year intervals. Lists of patients cared for by every general practitioner are kept by a committee which is responsible to the relevant Area Health Authority and these too have potential as a source of demographic information as well as of serving as a denominator for the calculation of ratios.

A corollary to the shortage of skilled staff at district level and to the necessity for immediately available data is that the quality of measurement and standards of design taught and expected by academics must be compromised. For instance, Cochrane (13) has very properly insisted that the randomized controlled trial is the only really acceptable way of improvement of health. But there can be no question of any but the most exceptional community physician ever performing a randomized controlled trial and even he will frequently find himself in the position of recommending the implementation of procedures which have not been properly evaluated by others. He must rely on the use of cruder methods for evaluating health services himself.

Problems

There are general principles underlying planning procedures which are universally applicable, but much of the detail is only applicable to the organization or system within which the plans are being formulated. In England there are widespread doubts as to how soon this will be generally available as and when it is needed. Clearly, to preach the need to practice epidemiology in a setting where the practitioner depends upon readily available information under such circumstances of doubt is to stretch credibility. A second problem, the availability of skilled manpower, has already been mentioned. The staff structure of the new NHS in support of the community physician, especially in the districts, is thin. Therefore, there is at the moment little prospect of more than somewhat meager routine information (a meagerness which despite some despondency one hopes will only be temporary), and little also of supplementing this to a significant extent with specially collected information.

We, the converted, have no doubt of the importance of epidemiology in the planning, management and evaluation of health services, but if we are to help to persuade skeptical colleagues to use it for this purpose we must be sure that the tools are available to do the job.

References

1. Joint Working Party on the Integration of Medical Work, *Community Medicine in Scotland,* Report of a Sub-Group on Community Medicine (Edinburgh: Her Majesty's Stationery Office, 1973). The new administrative structure is broadly similar in Scotland and Wales to that in England, but whereas in Scotland and Wales the interrelationship between the administrative subunits at the periphery and the larger units toward the center is hierarchical, in England it is not. For instance, although an Area Medical Officer (AMO) monitors the work of a District Community Physician (DCP), the AMO is not the DCP's "boss," nor for that matter is the Regional Medical Officer (RMO) the AMO's boss.

2. M. D. Warren, and R. M. Acheson, "Training in Community Medicine and Epidemiology," *International Journal of Epidemiology* 3 (1974), 275.

3. *Royal Commission on Medical Education* (London: Her Majesty's Stationery Office, 1969).

4. M. D. Warren, and R. M. Acheson, "Training in Community Medicine and Epidemiology in Britain," *International Journal of Epidemiology* 2 (1973), 371–78.

5. *Management and the Health Service,* eds. A. Gatherer and M. D. Warren (Oxford: Pergamon, 1971).

6. *Handbook in Community Medicine,* ed. A. Nelson (Bristol: E. & S. Livingstone, 1975).

7. J. N. Morris, *Uses of Epidemiology,* 3rd ed. (Edinburgh: E. & S. Livingstone, and Baltimore: Williams and Wilkins, 1975).

8. *Positions, Movements and Directions in Health Services Research,* ed. G. McLachlan (London: Oxford Univ. Press, 1975).

9. R. M. Acheson, "Epidemiology and the Community Physician," *Public Health* 89 (1975), 97–102.

10. Department of Health and Social Security, *Report of Working Party*

on *Medical Administrators* (London: Her Majesty's Stationery Office, 1972).

11. E. G. Knox, W. W. Holland, and J. N. Morris, "Planning Medical Information Systems in a Unified Health Service," *Lancet*, No. 7779 (1972), pp. 696–700.

12. J. Ashley, "Present State of Statistics from Hospital In-Patient Data and Their Uses," *British Journal of Preventive and Social Medicine* 26 (1972), 135–47.

13. A. L. Cochrane, *Effectiveness and Efficiency: Random Reflections on Health Services* (London: Nuffield Provincial Hospitals Trust, 1972).

8
JOHANNES MOSBECH, M.D.

HEALTH STATISTICS IN PLANNING SCANDINAVIAN HEALTH CARE

Introduction

Societies are changing more and more rapidly. So are their health care problems. Not many decades ago control of infectious diseases was the main subject of health statistics, but as these diseases declined we experienced an important change in disease patterns. Such chronic diseases as arteriosclerosis, coronary heart disease, diabetes mellitus, as well as accidents, suicides, and environmentally related diseases became the major focal issues. Health administrators and planners must have sufficient information to deal with this change and to count, register, and evaluate developments. Current vital statistical information is needed, but well planned ad hoc studies are often mandatory to elucidate specific problems. Epidemiologists are playing a role in identifying the nature and magnitude of problems and in bringing together medical and statistical expertise. To be successful those epidemiologists, statisticians, and health planners attached to either national or regional health statistical units or university departments of epidemiology have to work in close cooperation with the health authorities.

The National Health Service of Denmark has had its own health statistics unit for many years. Its original responsibility was the compilation of mortality statistics as well as statistics of infectious diseases. Its publications date back nearly a hundred years. The office still collects data on mortality and morbidity, but in recent years better use has been made of its information as its productivity extended beyond simple descriptions of the statistical data. The department has gradually changed into a health planning unit, where physicians with epidemiological knowledge work as a team with statisticians and health planners. This means that much more detailed input data is needed, not only about disease patterns, but also about resources, personnel, and costs involved in primary health care as well as hospital treatment, preventive activity as well as after-care, rehabilitation, and other extended care provisions.

Denmark, with five million inhabitants, has 750,000 admissions to hospitals every year, with 15 per cent of the population being admitted. Every year there are two million hospital outpatient consultations and, on the average, each citizen sees his general practitioner six times.

Planners have had to face the following general trends in the health services during the 1960's:

Aging of the population which led to use of half of all hospital beds by persons over sixty-five years of age;

Steadily rising costs of health services; in Denmark in 1971, 7.6 per cent of the gross national product was spent on health (in the United Kingdom the comparable figure was 4.7 per cent).

Relatively high costs of hospital-based care; during the 1960's there was a considerable expansion of hospital services with an increase in expenditures of 20 per cent per year, due to increases in personnel, buildings, and equipment. In 1972 there were 87 beds per 10,000 inhabitants. This expansion has been brought to an end and increasing stress put on primary health care given by general practitioners;

Environmental diseases have been uncovered in increasing numbers, and have amplified need and demand for preventive action;

Improved treatment measures have steadily increased the number of disabled persons in need of after-care and rehabilitation;

Improved medical technology has resulted in the establishment of specialized coronary care, dialysis, and other units, and a number of complicated surgical procedures like renal and heart transplantation, activities which have put a heavy burden on financial resources, and created an urgent demand for evaluation of all new procedures to establish priorities in these fields;

These and other changes in the health care system have had an impact on the number of physicians, nurses, and paramedical personnel needed; nationwide registration of medical personnel has become of the greatest importance;

Within the altered disease patterns a number have been recognized as specific and characteristic for modern industrialized society; among them are: myocardial infarction, lung cancer, traffic accidents, abortions, and abuse of drugs and alcohol.

Screening Programs

When the specific control problems faced by today's health authorities are considered, examples can be chosen to show how epidemiological information is helping administrators to make decisions. With growing interest in preventive medicine certain groups increasingly demand screening activities. Screening is a costly, time- and personnel-consuming exercise, and careful evaluation of its results is necessary before it can be brought into general use. Screening for cervical cancer was introduced following reports of positive results in British Columbia. But for ethical reasons it is extremely difficult to carry out the controlled trials necessary to evaluate the outcome of screening. Such controlled trials should compare groups screened with groups not screened, to show whether screening is of benefit. The fact that the mortality from cervical cancer has not changed more in the areas where screening has been introduced must give rise to some doubts concerning the justification for continuation of this activity.

Mass screening for pulmonary tuberculosis was established decades ago, but now the disease has declined considerably. In 1971, 850,000 persons were X-rayed, and only 140 cases of tuberculosis of the lungs were found in persons with specific exposure to the disease. The cost of finding a single case of lung tuberculosis was $15,000. Based on a careful epidemiological evaluation and cost-benefit analysis of the results of mass screening for tuberculosis, the Danish National Health Service decided to abandon mass screening for tuberculosis in 1973 and concentrate on screening of specific groups known to have high risk of infection.

Screening for asymptomatic urinary infection in pregnant women, which some consider a mechanism to prevent later chronic uremia, has been under consideration as a part of the health examination for pregnant women in Denmark. It will, however, not be introduced before it is carefully tested and evaluated in a controlled trial. The form of screening that consists of a series of laboratory tests carried out using an autoanalyzer, possibly combined with health examinations, is not felt to be justified by the health authorities, who have based their decision on all evidence currently available in Denmark. Vaccination programs play an important part in preventive medicine. The potential value of vaccination against measles has recently been investigated by asking in a postal questionnaire a representative sample of the population about the occurrence of the disease. The results gave the disease incidence, age distribution, complication rate, and these epidemiological data formed a useful base on which to decide whether a larger vaccination program would be justified.

Primary Health Care

The current trend in health services is, as mentioned above, toward an increased use of primary health care. There is, however, limited knowledge of work done in this area. An important Swedish study on the use of health services is worth mentioning. This is a person-based study which describes the age distribution of the patients, the diagnoses, their use of drugs, and so forth. During the three-month study, 18,000 physician consultations were registered, and 25,000 prescriptions were issued; in total, 47 per cent of the populations had some formal registered contact with their physicians. Epidemiological studies of this kind elucidate in a valuable way the demand to be met in the population by the health authorities. Studies of this kind are, however, cumbersome; it is difficult to obtain the data, even during a limited period of observation. Simple record forms are necessary, classification of diseases and treatment is often a problem, and data reduction is necessary in order to present the results in a form that is meaningful to health administrators.

Infectious diseases are on the decline. Two illustrations, however, show that important infectious disease problems can still arise. A fourfold increase of malaria has recently been reported in Denmark. An analysis has shown that it was due to increased travel by Danes to those areas where the disease is endemic, combined with insufficient prophylactic treatment, as well as an increased number of infected immigrants from Pakistan. These results are being published to alert the public as well as physicians. We have recently reported a considerable increase of hepatitis in Denmark, primarily serum infectious hepatitis affecting narcotics abusers. Careful registration of this notifiable disease has conditioned effective preventive efforts.

Hospital Care

Hospital data can be of specific value for health administrators, but the traditional formal information giving no more than the number of admissions with crude categories of diagnoses and treatment is of limited use. The introduction of computerized statistics based on hospital discharge abstracts with diagnosis, length of stay, manner of admission, state at discharge, as well as individual person number, and so forth, offers a wealth of information, invaluable for the planning and for the optimal use of the costly hospital sector. We have been using the information provided by hospital statistics about special categorical disease groups for planning specialized services (e.g., the department of hematology) in given areas of medical practice. The inclusion of data on use of hospital personnel and resources which is being planned will give the hospital statistics even greater value.

Sensible use of material of this kind can point to interesting differences, e.g., different lengths of stay in hospital for the same disease for comparable patient groups, which can only be changed once they are made known. A difficulty with hospital statistics in this form is the danger of "drowning" in paper; one responsibility of the epidemiologist is to make the material, which in itself has great research potential, a useful tool for hospital management in planning as well as in day-to-day operations. Some hospital departments are especially demanding of resources; renal dialysis units and coronary care units are examples. Based on an epidemiological analysis of the incidence of chronic uremia we have worked out a plan for the number of dialysis centers needed in Denmark: one unit per one million inhabitants; we have 28 patients per one million currently on dialysis (the United Kingdom has 21). The trend toward dialysis and transplantation is carefully monitored. It is important in this case to take into account the use of combined statistics. The 1960–71 mortality statistics show a 35–40 per cent decrease of terminal uremia in Denmark and Sweden. One could be tempted to think this due to the dialysis and transplantation activity, but decrease in glomerulonephritis due to decline of streptococcus infections, and decrease in nephropathy due to abuse of the analgesic phenacetine have probably been the primary determinants.

During the last few years we have seen an increase in the number of abortions due to a change in the law. The number of abortions has increased from about 12,000 to 20,000 (we have 70,000 births annually). When the law was introduced three years ago it was impossible to foresee its consequences. To meet the increased need for hospital service good current statistics and epidemiological evaluations of the trend had to be at hand.

Disease Registers

Registers can also be a useful epidemiological tool for planning purposes. A Cancer Registry on a national basis was introduced in Denmark thirty years ago. In its early days the register only accumulated epidemiological data which described the disease patterns, but now cancer registers are used for follow-up, giving cure rates as well as elucidating possible carcinogenic effects of environmental factors. The probable relation between cigarette smoking and lung cancer is an example; the possible relationship between working with PVC and liver cancer is another. It is important to use established registers for health evaluations and adapt them to serve the changing health problems of society. Epidemiological skill is needed to interpret the knowledge gained and to carry out the prospective studies often needed.

Myocardial infarction registers were established on the World Health Organization's initiative in a number of European countries and have yielded important information about etiological factors, treatment, and mortality. The specific value of these registers lies in their potential for patient follow-up. The registers are thus useful epidemiological research tools. The risk is, however, that overwhelming amounts of data are accumulated but never tabulated, analyzed, or interpreted. In some countries in Europe coronary heart disease registers have for this reason all been stopped or carried on with reduced amounts of data collection.

Mortality Statistics

Mortality statistics coded according to the International Classification of Disease (ICD) are longstanding and, although of limited value as a health indicator in developed societies, they are a valuable source of information. These statistics are based on the data given on death certificates and thus must be cautiously interpreted. The steep increase reported in mortality from asthma in young people which occurred in Great Britain as well as in other countries in the late 1960's is an example of the value of mortality statistics in pointing toward an important health hazard. Further studies have made it probable that overdoses from "Medihalers" were the cause of this increase. Widespread warnings about the high risks of overdosage resulted in rapid disappearance of this epidemic.

Mortality statistics in Scandinavian countries have shown a steep increase in mortality from liver cirrhosis during recent years, running parallel with the increased consumption of alcohol. Further study is being carried out on these cases, based on data from mortality statistics, to elucidate more detail about the etiological and epidemiological factors. A third example of use of mortality statistics is provided by the reports from different centers of a possible positive correlation between the softening of drinking water and mortality rates from ischemic heart disease. This raises the problem of whether soft drinking water per se is a health hazard. Further studies are needed, but at present the introduction of water softeners, recommended for industrial use, is being questioned for drinking water. Close cooperation between the epidemiologists, engineers, and health authorities is needed in this matter.

Epidemiology, Health Statistics, and Planning of Health Services

Many important health problems exist in our changing developed societies; careful descriptions of disease trends as well as evaluations of our preventive and curative activities are necessary. We must, based on the best available knowledge, find a balance between preventive measures and curative activity, between primary care and hospital treatment, and between the use of medical and paramedical staff. We have some knowledge of the etiology of diseases. For example, there is a strong positive correlation between cigarette smoking and lung cancer as well as coronary occlusion. Cigarette consumption was, until recently, increasing. The psychology of cigarette smoking is apparently so complex that it has been impossible to devise means to overcome this from the health information hitherto available. Traffic accidents have for long been a heavy burden; hospital and mortality statistics have shown an alarming increase, but the phenomenon has apparently been accepted as an inescapable cost of the further development of the society. It seemed that an oil crisis was necessary to change the overall situation. Increasing oil prices resulted in traffic speed limits which have cut morbidity and mortality rates by 30–40 per cent. Last year the lives of about 400 persons in Denmark were saved because of improved road traffic conditions. The examples quoted should show that satisfactory current statistics on disease patterns, morbidity, and mortality, as well as prevention and curative measures are most useful for planning purposes. Epidemiologists play a useful role as members of a team evaluating the statistics at hand and planning necessary projects for collection of specific information.

Finally, I would like to mention a practical form of cooperation in the

SCANDINAVIAN HEALTH CARE PLANNING121

health planning field which has been useful in our area. The NOMESKO (Scandinavian Committee for Medical Statistics) has played an important role in the development of meaningful and comparable health information in the Scandinavian countries during the last ten years. The committee was organized by the Nordic Council and members appointed by their own governments.

The committee consists of physicians, epidemiologists, health statisticians, health planners, and administrators, altogether some 30–40 persons, who meet regularly several times a year. Subgroups with ad hoc specialists on call deal with problems like birth registration, individual-based health registration, establishment of health information data bases, disease classifications, and so forth. Papers are presented and practical recommendations made of approaches which have been of value for descriptive analysis of demands and evaluation of procedures in the health field.

9

WALTER W. HOLLAND, M.D., AND SUSIE GILDERDALE

THE ROLE OF
HEALTH SERVICES RESEARCH
IN PLANNING FOR HEALTH
IN GREAT BRITAIN

Introduction

Until comparatively recently, the British National Health Service has been "planned" largely by a mixture of tradition and advocacy. New services have been introduced without proper evaluation, on the assumption that they would automatically improve outcome. Existing services have continued for no better reason than that they have always existed. There has been resistance to, and suspicion of, health services research from many health administrators and clinicians who prefer to put their faith in experience in the field, instinct, and intelligent guesswork. "The traditional dominance of the physical sciences has tended toward a partial view of research activity . . ." (1).

But whether we like it or not health, or lack of it, is big business. The Health Service in Britain employs one in every thirty of our work force and accounts for about a tenth of all public expenditures (2). And thus, questions of efficiency and the best use of increasingly limited resources are relevant and must be scientifically investigated.

In the reorganization of the United Kingdom's National Health Service which took effect in April 1974, greater emphasis was placed on the importance of proper planning, based on research findings, for the improvement and development of health care services. The fundamental unit in the planning process is the Area. The Area Health Authority plans for its smaller communities or districts, and has a strong influence on the allocation of national resources. The main operational policies are put into effect by the District Management Team who, with the Health Care Planning Team, commission and make use of research findings in their assessment of how best to deploy resources. The aim of this paper is to outline briefly some of the problems at the interface of research and planning, to give examples of two main strands of health services research, and finally to discuss the implementation of research findings and the role of the epidemiologist in deciding priorities.

Research and Administration: The Need for Compromise

One of the problems in health planning is the different, and often conflicting, approaches of the research worker and the administrator or policy-maker. This has been discussed fully elsewhere (3, 4) but it may be helpful to summarize the main points here. It is basically a conflict between the particular and the general. From the administrator's standpoint, the view is general; he must decide what to do and how to do it. He often has inadequate information on which to base his decisions but he has to decide. The research worker, on the other hand, works on the particulars—breaking down and defining a problem precisely—and looking for a specific answer to a specific question. There are time scale differences as well. Accurate information may be required before an urgent policy can be put into effect and this may widen the gulf between the administrator who must have quick results and the research worker who is reluctant to carry out a hurried and possibly unsatisfactory study.

A compromise can only be based on improved understanding on both sides. The administrator must realize that a research problem has to be rigorously defined before it can be adequately investigated. The research worker must accept that the administrator has to answer general questions in some fashion, and he must therefore indicate whether and how his findings can safely and productively be generalized. The research worker and the administrator must therefore try to choose a *specific* research problem which can provide the solution to a *general* question. And health services research must try to answer realistic questions formulated at a time when they can affect policy or help decide priorities in health.

Research and Policy: Some Examples

Various studies undertaken by the Social Medicine and Health Services Research Unit at St. Thomas's Hospital Medical School were occasioned by questions of local or national policy, and we would like to consider six of these here.

The Lambeth Studies.

The Lambeth Studies (5) centered around the policy problems of planning the services of a hospital group to meet the needs of the local community. The general question was, "If St. Thomas's is to be responsible for providing total hospital care for the community, what hospital facilities are needed?" It was clearly an impossible task to measure all needs; the research approach was to use a number of indicator conditions, measure their prevalence in the community, and then make an assessment of unmet need in terms of hospital services.

Four indicator conditions were chosen to illustrate different types of health care:

Cardiorespiratory disease which represents about 60 per cent of all mortality in London;

Functional disability which leads to major use of community and hospital resources;

Skin disease which is a major component of outpatient and general practitioner care;

Peptic ulceration which is a common cause of illness both in general practice and in hospital.

The prevalence of each of these conditions in a random sample of the population was measured and the associated use of health services determined. The findings indicated that there were sufficient hospital resources available for cardiorespiratory disease, skin disease, and peptic ulceration but that those with functional disability were inadequately covered.

The Frimley Studies.

The studies in Frimley were designed to answer a specific policy question in connection with the building of a new "best buy" hospital. The idea behind this was to provide fewer acute hospital beds per 1,000 population than the norm, with more diagnostic and treatment facilities linked to comprehensive community services, the emphasis being placed on high bed turnover and a policy of community care. We undertook two main studies to test the validity and examine the consequences of this policy.

The first was a randomized controlled trial of early discharge from hospital following operations for two simple surgical conditions, hernia and varicose veins (6). Most general practitioners and all three surgeons in the area agreed to cooperate, and patients with these conditions who were considered suitable, either for the normal seven-day stay in a hospital or for discharge after 48 hours, were allocated at random to one or the other duration group. The effect of early discharge in terms of clinical outcome and of the social, psychological, and economic impact on the patient, the family and the health service, were assessed. There was no difference in clinical outcome for hernia patients discharged after 48 hours. Varicose vein patients discharged early did have more complications than those who stayed in hospital for seven days, but the complications were relatively trivial. Early discharge was more acceptable to the patient than staying in a hospital for the longer period. The economic consequences of early discharge have not yet been fully worked out but there does not seem to be any great difference in total cost between the two procedures.

The second study in Frimley concerned the care of stroke patients in the area (7). A register of stroke patients was established and all forms of hospital and community care for this condition examined. Briefly, the findings indicated that about one-third of these patients died within three weeks of the stroke. After three months, more than half of the survivors were functioning as they had done before the stroke. This finding is obviously of some importance in the organization and planning of services for this condition and suggests that to create special stroke rehabilitation units at great expense is not a good use of resources since few patients would benefit. A high proportion of stroke survivors will regain their former functions with normal medical care, as was the case in Frimley where there were no special facilities.

Basingstoke Studies.

The expansion of the area in and around Basingstoke after its designation as a new town meant that the existing medical services were inadequate to meet the rapidly growing demand. Those involved in the planning of medical care were anxious to establish an integrated health care system and to use Basingstoke as a prototype for new health care ideas in the future. There were a number of problems to be examined and we would like to look briefly at two of these.

First, in the psychiatric field, it seemed likely that some form of community care would develop; at the time of these studies, the traditional mental hospital was the only major provider of care for the mentally ill, and clinical information suggested that there were long-stay patients who could function adequately outside the hospital. But selection of patients suitable for life in the community is notoriously difficult since no single individual can know the precise abilities of large numbers of long-stay patients. A study of functional ability in about 1,000 such patients has provided a possible tool for this selection (8).

The second research problem was to decide what sort of hospital care could be provided for patients without removing them from the supervision of their general practitioner. For this purpose a study was carried out of patients admitted to the hospital under the care of their own general practitioner, compared with those admitted under consultant care. Patients admitted under GP care were found to be in more terminal stages of illness and to require far fewer diagnostic facilities than those under consultant care. Thus, although GPs and consultants tended to admit the same diagnostic mix of patients, they were using inpatient beds for different types of care. This has obvious policy implications in a situation where general practitioners can care for their patients in hospital.

National Study of Health and Growth.
Changes in government policy can pose questions for the research worker. A clear and recent example of this is the withdrawal of free school milk, which provided the opportunity to assess the influence of these factors on the growth of schoolchildren. In this study, height, weight, skinfold thickness and a number of other variables are being measured over a period of years in a sample of schoolchildren in 28 areas of England and Scotland. These are a stratified random sample, weighted to include more of the poorer areas. The study is designed to assess changes in growth patterns and detect possible effects of changes in social or economic policy, such as the withdrawal of free school milk. Preliminary results indicate that the method is feasible and yields reproducible results. Initial investigation of the results of the first two years of study suggest that there are major differences in the height and weight of children from different social class groups on entry to school and that these persist throughout schooling. Though school milk may minimally increase growth rate during school years, the large social class gap already evident on school entry suggests that early intervention is most likely to be beneficial.

Screening Study.
For many years there has been public demand for the introduction of screening, and for methods of early detection of disease to be developed in the United Kingdom. But there is still no concrete evidence that screening is worthwhile. In an effort to shed some light in this area, particularly in relation to the multiphasic screening of middle-aged individuals, a controlled trial of multiphasic screening in two large group practices in South-East London is being undertaken. Patients aged between forty and sixty-four years registered with these practices have been randomly allocated to two groups, one receiving periodic screening, the other normal clinical care. Results so far show little, if any difference in mortality or level of function between the control and the screened group five years after initial screening. It is possible, however, that there may be a difference in terms of combined coronary risk factors between the control and screened group in young middle-aged men. The implication of this is that screening merely makes people more aware of their risk of developing a particular disease and encourages them to modify their behavior. It may thus be more productive to concentrate on reducing risk factors, such as smoking and overweight, rather than to introduce screening and try to develop early treatment by pharmacological means.

Responaut Study.
A final example of research occasioned by policy was the study of the possibility of life in the community for responaut patients (9). The origin of this investigation was the political decision to find out whether very severely disabled patients could be cared for in their own homes and what consequences this would have. The study was based on a very small number of patients but it has shown that patients with such severe disabilities can be cared for at home at a cost similar to that of hospital care. This has led to a change in policy at least in the St. Thomas's Health District which has now decided on a home care policy for such patients, wherever possible.

Research and Priorities: Two Examples

One of the major tasks in health service administration and research is to decide how best to allocate limited resources; whether, for example, to spend more on hospital or preventive services, to intervene in the disease process, or to treat a particular condition. For this kind of planning adequate data are needed and these can best be obtained by means of descriptive epidemiological or medical care studies. The following are two examples of this kind of work.

Respiratory Studies. The first is concerned with the development of chronic respiratory disease. Studies of chronic respiratory disease in children in Kent and Harrow (10, 11) have suggested the importance of events in childhood on the further development of chronic respiratory disease in older children and young adults. These studies appear to indicate that:

Respiratory infections in the first year of life are important in influencing levels of ventilatory function and frequency of disease in later life;

Children who develop respiratory infection and symptoms in their early years have more symptoms, more disease, and lower levels of ventilatory function in later years;

The frequency of respiratory infections in the first year of life are influenced by the smoking habits of parents; the children of parents who smoke have more respiratory infections in the first year of life than those whose parents do not smoke;

Children who smoke have more symptoms of respiratory disease and more illnesses than children who do not smoke;

Children who live in polluted urban areas have more disease and lower levels of ventilatory function than children who live in unpolluted areas.

These findings suggest that to prevent chronic respiratory disease it is essential to intervene early. The most important factor in the disease process appears to be cigarette smoking. Influencing the smoking habits of young children and their parents may be crucial in preventing the development of respiratory disease in later life, and thus in improving subsequent mortality and reducing the consumption of health services resources.

Studies in General Practice. The second example of descriptive work is seen in the studies in general practice (12–15). These were undertaken with the aim of examining the content of the general practitioner's work, and of trying to determine what influences the demand for primary care services. These studies have demonstrated the differences in the patterns of disease presenting in primary care and in the hospital, and the types of personnel and facilities required for care within the primary health care center. They have also shown that most people visit the general practitioner because of physical disease and not, as many have tended to assume, for psychological treatment. We do not yet have any clear idea as to the factors that influence demand. But it is apparent that only about one in thirty symptom events lead to consultation with a general practitioner, and that individuals or families who are high demanders of service in one year are not necessarily high demanders in subsequent years.

Implementation of Research Findings

It would be difficult to overestimate the importance of implementation; it is, after all, one of the main reasons for carrying out health services research. But it is not easy and there are no good precedents, and this brings us back to the relationship between the research worker and the administrator which is the key to making research relevant and therefore worth implementing.

At St. Thomas's we have attempted to establish a close relationship in two ways. First, one senior administrator, who is primarily responsible to the district administrator, is specifically concerned with examining research and seeing how it can be applied. Second, the director of the Research Unit is a member of the District Management Team which is responsible for the delivery of health services. These strong links between research and planning make the implementation of research findings a practical possibility since the administrator is involved in the research process and the research worker in the planning process. And only by this kind of cooperation can health services research hope to provide the basis for improved health care which is surely its ultimate aim.

In conclusion, a word of caution on the role of the epidemiologist in deciding priorities. That he should play an important part in decision-making is beyond question. He must help to interpret available information, assess its validity and applicability, and provide guidance on the relative merits of different methods of care for the same group of patients. But in the assessment of priorities in a situation where two different services are competing for resources, the epidemiologist is no better placed than any other member of the decision-making team to make what is essentially a value judgment.

References

1. D. A. K. Black, "Organization of Health Services Research," *British Medical Bulletin* 30(1974), 199–202.

2. Andrew Creese, "Economics and Health Service Planning," *Social Medicine and Health Services Research Unit Annual Report 1973–74,* (London: St. Thomas's Hospital Medical School), pp. 117–28.

3. W. W. Holland and J. W. Owen, "A Conflict of Roles," *Health and Social Service Journal* 84 (1974), 609.

4. J. W. Owen and W. W. Holland, "Research and Administration in Health—The Uneasy Relationship," in *A Monograph on Planning for Health Services* (London: King Edward's Hospital Fund for London, 1975).

5. W. W. Holland and J. J. Waller, "Population Studies in the London Borough of Lambeth," *Community Medicine* 126 (1971), 153.

6. M. W. Adler, J. J. Waller, et al., "A Randomized Controlled Trial of Early Discharge for Inguinal Hernia and Varicose Veins: Some Problems of Methodology," *Medical Care* 12 (1974), 541–47.

7. J. M. Weddell, "Strokes—A Medico-Social Problem," in *The Skandia International Symposium on Rehabilitation after Central Nervous System Trauma (CNST)* (Stockholm: n.p., 1973), pp. 25–27.

8. M. Clarke, J. J. Waller, and B. Webster, "The Assessment and Progress of Long-Stay and Elderly Psychiatric Patients: The Predictive Validity of a Ward Behaviour Questionnaire," *British Journal of Psychiatry* 127 (1975) 149.

9. K. Dunnell, M. W. Adler, et al., "Collaboration Between Health and Social Services: A Study of the Care of Responauts," *Community Medicine* 218 (1972), 503.

10. W. W. Holland, et al., "Indications for Measures to Be Taken in Childhood to Prevent Chronic Respiratory Disease," *Milbank Memorial Fund Quarterly* 47 (1969), 215.

11. W. W. Holland, et al., "Factors Influencing the Onset of Chronic Respiratory Disease," *British Medical Journal* 2 (1969), 205.

12. D. C. Morrell, H. G. Gage, and N. A. Robinson, "Patterns of Demand in General Practice," *Journal of the Royal College of General Practitioners* 21 (1971), 331.

13. D. C. Morrell, "Symptom Interpretation in General Practice," *Journal of the Royal College of General Practitioners* 22 (1972), 297.

14. D. C. Morrell, H. G. Gage, and N. A. Robinson, "Referral to Hospital by General Practitioners," *Journal of the Royal College of General Practitioners* 21 (1971), 77.

15. D. C. Morrell, H. G. Gage, and N. A. Robinson, "Symptoms in General Practice," *Journal of the Royal College of General Practitioners* 21 (1971), 32.

10
BASIL S. HETZEL, M.D.

A MODEL FOR PUBLIC LEARNING IN HEALTH CARE: ADMINISTRATIVE APPLICATIONS OF EPIDEMIOLOGY AND HEALTH STATISTICS IN AUSTRALIA

Introduction

My approach to this problem out of Australian experience reflects the current health situation of what has been called "The Lucky Country." We certainly have great material benefits: a land mass, nearly as great as the United States, full of mostly untapped minerals and oil; a population 6 per cent the size of that of the United States which experiences only minor race problems by contrast to that country; a government, as in the United States and Canada, divided between federal and state jurisdictions (usually in conflict!); founded after the American Revolution, Australia remains part of the British Commonwealth. The health care system resembles that of the United States and Canada. There are many subsystems: Repatriation (Veterans), Pensioner (Social Security), private care, public hospital, and community programs. But private care is predominantly financed by a Voluntary Health Insurance System composed of over 100 separate funds. Over 40 per cent of the licensed medical practitioners receive salaries, mostly within the public hospital, state, and federal health departments. Politically, however, the interests of private practitioners are dominant.

The recent situation was one of considerable turmoil and questioning following the election of a federal Labor (social democratic) Government in December 1972. This government was pledged to major health policy initiatives in the fields of community health care and health insurance. These have been resisted by the organized medical profession along the same lines of protest previously raised in other countries. The movement to preserve the freedom of the patient to choose his doctor and of the doctor to choose (and charge) his patient has been vigorously assisted by an unscrupulous mass media campaign which has adversely affected the image of the medical profession in Australia.

In the current controversies there has been some reference to epidemiological data and health statistics. The number of people not covered by health insurance (one million of a population of thirteen million) has been acknowledged by both political parties. A lack of facilities for the aged and chronically disabled has been highlighted. In such a situation, which after all obtains in many countries where health and health services have become a controversial issue, what is the value and appropriate use of epidemiological data and health statistics by the health administrator?

Before we can answer these and related questions, we need a model of how epidemiological data are being used within the social system. More particularly, we need a model of how changes come about and their relation, if any, to epidemiological data. I shall illustrate from Australian experience, but I believe the model presented may be appropriate for the United States.

I have been stimulated in my thinking by Donald Schon's book *Beyond the Stable State* (1), though it will not be possible in this space to develop his ideas at any length. However, we are experiencing in Australia at present a period of rapid social change during which a number of innovations in health care are taking place. These innovations offer an interesting series of examples of what Schon has called "public learning." They present case studies which I hope may be of some interest to health administrators in the United States. I have used them to derive a provisional model for public learning in the health care field.

Health information is the basic fuel which keeps the model going or the health care system in operation. Without health information public learning is not possible. But of course public learning is going on all the time with whatever information is available. At present in the United States, a recent study shows, the major source of health information, other than the doctor, is television commercials. I believe the same would be true of Australia. Can we wonder at a certain lack of understanding of basic health issues? There is an urgent need not only for the collection and analysis, but also the dissemination of health information

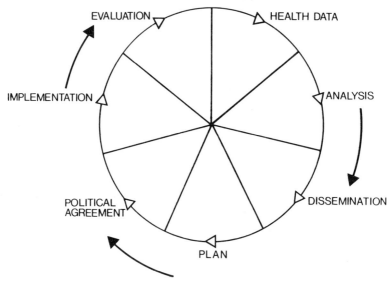

Figure 10–1. A Model for Public Learning.

in the Western world today. I have written a Penguin paperback, *Health and Australian Society* (2), to try to alleviate the situation in Australia.

A Model for Public Learning

The suggested model can be usefully represented by a wheel composed of a series of seven segments, as in Figure 10–1. The process begins with the collection of *health data* which may include mortality and morbidity data as well as information on usage and performance of health services. The next step is *analysis* and careful consideration of the meaning of the data. The third segment involves *dissemination,* not only through the scientific community but even more important through mass media to the community at large. Eventually a *plan* emerges from discussion between the epidemiologists, administrators, and other professionals involved. This plan then has to receive *political agreement* which often requires community consultation with the various groups involved. Eventually *implementation* can take place following the achievement of political agreement. Then after implementation, *evaluation* must occur which involves the collection of more data to provide the basis for review of the plan and inevitable modification in the light of experience.

Let us now consider five examples from the contemporary Australian health scene to illustrate this process of public learning:

Compulsory seat belt legislation;

Aboriginal health care;

Community health programs;

Compulsory health insurance;

Life style and health.

In the first case the rapid collection of epidemiological data has largely resolved public controversy. In the case of aboriginal health the epidemiological data indicate such a disaster that no serious public controversy exists regarding the health program; the problem is one of implementation and evaluation. In the case of community health programs and compulsory health insurance there is continuing controversy about the policies and plans being pursued, particularly involving the organized medical professional groups. In the fifth example the public learning process has been mainly influenced by mass media providing information destructive to health.

Seat Belt Legislation

The adoption of legislation requiring the compulsory wearing of seat belts is an Australian first in the Western world. It dates from the activities in the State of Victoria (population 3.5 million) of the Road Trauma Committee of the Royal Australasian College of Surgeons, and the activities of other interested bodies such as the Australian Medical Association and the Royal Automobile Club of Victoria (representing 500,000 motorists). Surgeons, daily faced with the effects of traffic accidents, had decided in the light of available data from Sweden and the United States (Stages 1 and 2) that compulsory wearing of seat belts (not just the provision of seat belts) was necessary to reduce this carnage. They initiated a mass media campaign particularly through the press in May 1970 (Stage 3). The Victorian State Parliamentary Select Committee on Road Safety (bipartisan) accepted the recommendation (Stage 4). In the face of mounting pressure assisted by a series of disastrous weekends on Victorian roads it was adopted by the State Government in November 1970 and became law in 1971 (Stages 5 and 6). Since that time there has been a significant fall in deaths and a fall in the numbers of accident victims presenting with head and facial injuries to hospitals (Stage 7; see Table 10–1). The wheel has therefore come full circle (Figure 10–2) with successful completion of each stage.

Table 10–1. Effect of Compulsory Seat Belt Legislation Victoria, Australia—1971*

Occupant Fatalities	1970	1971	Percentage change	P
Victoria	564	464	−17.7	<0.01
Rest of Australia	1426	1429	+ 0.2	
Occupant Injuries				
Victoria	14620	12454	−14.8	<0.01
Rest of Australia	39980	40396	+ 1.0	

* First nine months.
Source: Reference 3.

Since 1970 this legislation has quickly been adopted by the other states of Australia and is now gradually spreading to other countries. It indicates the role of the medical profession, the mass media, and the politician and the necessity of concerted action in order to bring about change in the light of epidemiological data. The health administrator was required to respond to these initiatives and to assist in taking the necessary steps including especially the collection of data for evaluation.

More recently, legislation requiring the compulsory collection of blood samples for alcohol determination from all traffic casualties coming to hospitals has been implemented in the states of Victoria and South Australia. But there have been difficulties in organization, administration, and making the data available which have not yet been overcome. This new initiative will eventually provide definitive information on the significance of alcohol consumption in relation to traffic accidents. At present, 5–10 per cent of the casualties (including drivers, passengers, and pedestrians) have grossly elevated levels (in excess of 0.15 per cent) (4). These data will require new initiatives in the setting up of treatment and rehabilitation services for heavy drinkers at a much

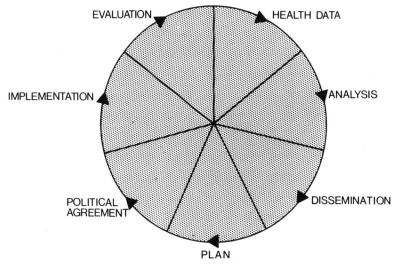

Figure 10–2. Seat Belt Legislation.

earlier stage in their drinking careers, with a correspondingly greater chance of success. So far, however, the cycle has barely got beyond the first segment.

Aboriginal Health

Health statistics on the Australian aboriginal population were not available until the late 1960's. Infant mortality data were first published in 1969 (Table 10–2). There is no specific recording of aboriginal race on the death certificate so these data were gained from the full-blood aboriginal population of the Northern Territory who could be identified by name. The infant mortality rate of 131 per 1,000 was a truly horrifying figure which was widely publicized. Two national seminars were held. The first, under government auspices, took place at the end of 1970 and the second at Monash University in May 1972. The first was concerned with traditional scientific and research investigation; the second with the total life situation of the people. Health was seen as part of the life situation of the aboriginal people and the cultural breakdown arising from contact with the white man since he arrived on the Australian continent in 1788. In contrast to the first, the

Table 10–2. Comparative Infant Mortality Rates (Deaths in the First Year per 1,000 Live Births)

Northern Territory Aborigines (full blood) (1965–67)	131.0
Australia (1958–60)	20.7
N.Z. Maori (1958–60)	51.0
U.S. Indian (1959)	47.0
South Africa (colored) (1959)	120.6
India (rural) (1958–59)	145.9

Source: Reference 5.

second seminar was attended by twenty aborigines of a total of seventy participants from all parts of Australia. These participants included aboriginal leaders and field workers along with anthropologists, sociologists, administrators, doctors, and public health nurses from the white community. In spite of considerable tension in the aboriginal group, a series of recommendations was accepted unanimously. These affirmed the integrity of the aboriginal people and the need to foster aboriginal community leadership. The health situation was seen as a community problem arising from cultural breakdown due to contact with European society. It required a comprehensive strategy aimed at drastic improvement in education, housing, and employment opportunities as well as health services. The implications were then spelled out in terms of setting up of a National Advisory Body representative of aboriginal, government, and nongovernment interests to advise on suitable programs. The need was recognized for special attention to health education, control of alcohol consumption, and family planning programs to be undertaken on the initiative of the local aboriginal communities themselves. The progress of such programs would be monitored by the collection of appropriate statistical information. The seminar recommended the keeping of separate health statistics for aborigines to enable suitable monitoring to occur (6).

Copies of these resolutions were sent to all members of both Houses of the Federal Parliament in Canberra. This certainly aroused interest. Then the election of a new Labor Government at the end of 1972 was followed by a major new thrust with the acceptance of the total cultural and ecological approach. This was in contrast to the previous fragmented

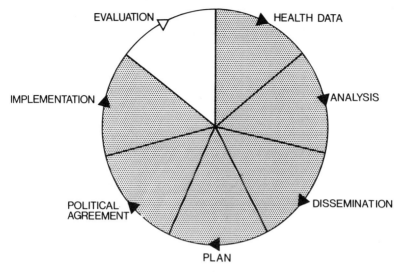

Figure 10–3. Aboriginal Health Care.

approach which relied largely on treatment services. A new division of Aboriginal Health was set up in the Federal Department of Health with an expert Advisory Committee including aboriginal representatives. New programs are under way including the training of aboriginal health assistants and community development projects.

Reverting to our wheel (Figure 10–3), following collection, analysis and dissemination of the data, the development of a plan for such a complex problem was greatly assisted by an interdisciplinary seminar which involved the aborigines themselves and was held on neutral ground in a university. Political acceptance by a newly elected vigorous government ensured rapid implementation of pilot projects which now require evaluation. The implications of the statistics could only be realized by a new Division of Aboriginal Health which has since taken over virtually complete responsibility for aboriginal health in all states except Queensland. This major administrative change was necessary to face the problem; it required political intervention and could not have occurred without it. I must pay tribute to the adaptability of many of the health administrators in this instance. However, there has inevitably been a lot of conflict. A complete change from the paternalism of senior health professionals in the past could not be expected from all. An unstable situation is going to continue, but the cycle already described still applies and offers the model for future strategy. This story follows in many respects the sequence of events leading up to the change in approach to the health of American Indians dating from 1955.

Community Health Programs

There has been increasing recognition of the importance of the development of better integrated and more comprehensive community health services to enable a better approach to be made to alteration of the pattern of modern morbidity as revealed by epidemiological data. In Australia various morbidity surveys have been carried out (2, 7) indicating the high prevalence of chronic illness and disability and mental illness and the close link between health and welfare needs. There was much interest in the model of the community health center as developed in the United Kingdom and also in the United States. A working party (of which I was a member) was set up in 1970 by the Australian Medical Association. In 1972 it published a report entitled "General Practice and Its Future in Australia" (8). This report was by no means radical: indeed, a reviewer in England described it as containing "remarkably few new ideas." However, in 1972 it was totally rejected in the most violent terms by the A.M.A. State Councils and by many rank and file members.

The election of the Labor government at the end of 1972 led to the setting up of a new National Hospitals and Health Services Commission which immediately pursued an active policy of initiating community health center development in all states. This policy met with considerable opposition in most states, which led to modification of the original proposals to better match local conditions of private general practice. My own experience in initiating a community health center comprising a team of allied health professionals providing domiciliary services has been quite traumatic but others have fared even worse. The situation has slowly improved with patience and acceptance of the need for time to evolve a suitable modus vivendi for Australian conditions. The National Commission has now recognized the need for modification of planning to take into account local conditions, a good example of the center–periphery problem described so well by Donald Schon.

Reverting to our cycle (Figure 10–4), the development of a plan appropriate to meet the situation revealed by modern medical morbidity was followed by political acceptance. However, the plan when implemented was resisted strongly by local groups so that modification had to occur. A number of pilot projects have now been established and evaluation measures are being set up with a view to early modification in the

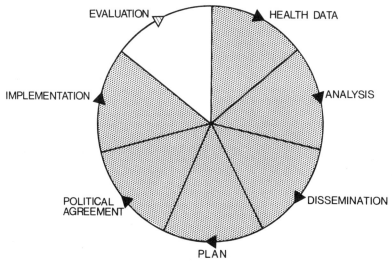

Figure 10–4. Community Health Programs.

light of the findings. One important feature of these community health projects is the involvement of the local community. We, as a university department of social and preventive medicine, have now assisted a number of local communities in the collection of data in order to prepare submissions for grants from the National Hospitals and Health Services Commission. The preparation of such submissions involves community consultation as well as the collection of data. Such consultation has not always occurred so that major conflicts have erupted later even after funds have been allotted for projects.

Compulsory Health Insurance

The next example of the application of health statistics is the development of the Compulsory Health Insurance Scheme for Australia. This plan was accepted as policy by the Labor party prior to its election and is now being implemented in the face of considerable opposition. It followed an official inquiry in 1969 by a committee, under the chairmanship of Mr. Justice Nimmo, appointed by the previous government. The inquiry revealed the inadequacies of the current voluntary health insurance scheme. The new scheme provides for universal entitlement for benefits (independent of a means test), covering basic hospital care and all medical services (9). It is to be financed by a separate health insurance fund administered by a statutory Commonwealth Health Insurance Commission. Finance will be derived mainly from revenues. The operation of the compulsory health insurance scheme would largely, though not completely, replace the operation of the Voluntary Health Insurance Funds, which would continue the coverage of private care. There would be encouragement of "bulk billing" by medical practitioners to minimize administrative costs. This scheme is being strongly opposed by the organized medical profession as well as the Voluntary Insurance Funds. These groups regard the scheme to be essentially one for "nationalization of the medical profession." For these reasons there has been a lack of responsible and constructive consultation between the government, the medical profession, and the Voluntary Health Insurance Funds, that is, the carriers. A series of explanatory seminars (on neutral ground as in the case of aboriginal health) would possibly have been useful in attempting to catalyze the process of change as well as in leading to some modification of the plan to meet existing conditions. A number of concessions have been made by the government but only after considerable mass media pressure, which does not help future negotiations. However, major conflict was probably inevitable in such a controversial issue. The scheme, now called "Medibank," still has to be implemented. At the time the Labor government was pushing ahead with a view to starting "Medibank" on July 1, 1975. So far, it has been accepted by only two states out of six, Tasmania and South Australia, with a third, Queensland, expected to join shortly. There are formidable difficulties and the phase in the cycle of public learning remains behind that of the community health center program: before rather than after implementation (Figure 10–5). It seems likely that considerable modification of the central plan will occur in different states. Indeed, the success of the scheme may well depend on the flexibility of the Health Insurance Commission.

It is not surprising that the manner of organization and financing of health services is so controversial in countries with private entrepreneural systems of practice. Large sums of money are involved. But the present fees received by doctors in Australia are largely (>50 per cent) derived from taxation revenue. This makes accountability and supervision an essential and inescapable result of the complexities of modern medicine. New strategies are, however, required by health administrators to assist change. Consultations on neutral ground need to be held to broaden the rather narrow views of participants committed to the special interests of the institution to which they belong, be it a private or government body. The alternative is polarization, confrontation via

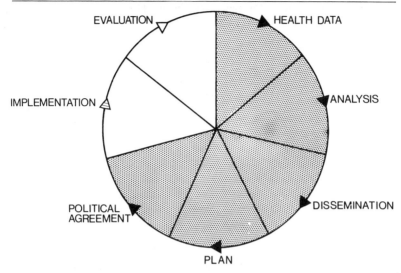

Figure 10–5. Compulsory Health Insurance.

the mass media with destructive effects on future negotiations and the likelihood of a constructive outcome. However, confrontation may be unavoidable and may be necessary for a satisfactory resolution of conflict. It may be that we are going to have much more confrontation in the future than in the past. In these circumstances, reliable health information constitutes the only objective input.

Future Policies: Life Style and Health

If we really took our health statistics seriously, particularly mortality data, we would be more concerned with other issues than simply health services and health finance. International comparison of age-specific mortality is readily made between countries following the ICD classification and at a similar stage of social development. Australia, New Zealand, and Canada have very similar figures for age-specific mortality at all ages (10). These are significantly higher than the figures for England and Wales although similar to those of Scotland. They are much higher than the figures for Sweden and Holland. Similar trends are evident in age-specific mortality due to heart disease (Table 10–3), and the same is true for accidents, poisoning, and violence.

Table 10-3. Age-Specific Mortality (Deaths Per 100,000)
Due to Heart Disease—1971

	35–44 years	45–54 years	55–64 years
Australia	77	277	848
Canada	57	217	631
England and Wales	66	240	689
Scotland	85	314	882
Sweden	37	142	493
Holland	43	164	482

Source: Reference 10.

The reasons for these differences are multiple. However, it seems likely that the major reason is not in the health services, which are well developed in all these countries, as much as in variations in life style (2). This is indicated particularly by the marked differences in death rates due to accidents, poisoning, and violence (Table 10-4). The characteristics of different life styles such as alcohol consumption, cigarette smoking, and awareness of health hazards are important areas which

Table 10-4. Age-Specific Mortality (Deaths Per 100,000)
Due to Accidents, Poisoning, and Violence—1971

	<1 year	1–4 years	5–14 years	15–24 years	25–34 years
Australia	64	33	19	90	66
Canada	95	35	25	84	70
England and Wales	58	21	13	39	30
Scotland	159	27	18	47	39
Sweden	14	12	14	54	51
Holland	47	33	20	46	36

Source: Reference 10.

should have more attention from health administrators than they have had in the past. The importance of health education (motivation so that health information is used to modify life style) in the United States health scene has been pointed out by a former Surgeon-General (11).

At this stage, we are primarily concerned with health information as a basis for necessary improvements in health and health services. What, then, are the existing sources of health information? In a recent survey of sources of health information in the United States, 85 per cent of those surveyed said they looked to their physicians and to one other source for health information. The other source was television commercials! In 1973, Steinfeld states that of the $80 billion spent on health in the United States, 92 per cent was for health care, a little over 4 per cent for biomedical research, 3 per cent was for such public health measures as immunization, purification of water supplies and sewage treatment, and less than 0.5 per cent was spent on health information.

Reverting to our model (Figure 10–6), the cycle has hardly proceeded beyond the first two stages in Australia as far as authentic information is concerned. It is obvious that future developments in health and health care require a much better level of health information for the community at large. At present there is widespread ignorance, reflected by general apathy. Health is, however, becoming a more important political issue. One important function of the health administrator is to see that a much better level of health information is provided for the public. If this were achieved television commercials would not be so influential, especially among the younger generation. Better health information should produce a more enlightened electorate from which, indirectly, more enlightened political decisions will finally come.

Conclusion

A model indicating the relationship between health statistics and change in the health care system has been developed in the light of recent Australian experience. A series of major innovations have been reviewed, involving the introduction of legislation making the wearing of seat belts compulsory, a new approach to the health of the Australian aboriginal people, a new community health program, and the introduction of compulsory health insurance. Each of these innovations is at a different stage in the following nine-step basic cycle:

the collection of health information;

the analysis of health information;

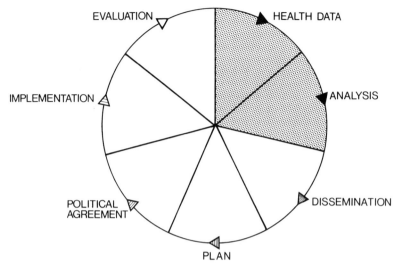

Figure 10–6. Life Style and Health.

the dissemination of health information through mass media and education programs;

the planning of new health care programs in the light of this information;

the presentation of plans for consideration by the community and its representatives;

the achievement of a consensus on change;

the implementation of change;

the evaluation of the change;

the modification of the program in the light of evaluation.

The health administrator may be active at all points in this process. However, he need not be involved at all stages all the time. It is his job to facilitate the process of public learning by the involvement of the whole community to which he is responsible. Discontinuities in the process of public learning are bound to occur; the administrator is required to be flexible, an uncommon quality not always easy to maintain with ongoing responsibility for a health service.

However, the changing nature of man's health problems and the impact of new technologies may change the rules of the game in health administration. The present lag in the application of new knowledge so characteristic of Western countries including, I believe, the United States, is well put by Donald Schon when he describes United States government departments as "a series of memorials to past problems" (1). The only way to prepare for change is through the establishment of an adequate health information system. However, beyond this is the need to accept a process for the analysis and use of health information along the lines suggested in this model. This process involves publicity, planning, and consultation before and after planning, political agreement, implementation, and evaluation. At all stages health information including epidemiological data is vital, and the only final resource for the resolution of the conflicts which will inevitably arise. Acceptance of such a model by high level administrators and politicians would do much to facilitate necessary change and would diminish the cost and waste arising as a byproduct of the inertia of the present system.

References

1. D. A. Schon, *Beyond the Stable State* (London: Maurice Temple Smith Ltd., 1971).

2. B. S. Hetzel, *Health and Australian Society* (Australia: Penguin Books, 1974).

3. P. Vulcan, "Australia's Safety Belt Use Laws: The Results of the Law," *Proceedings, National Safety Belt Usage Conference* (Washington, D.C.: National Highway Traffic Safety Administration, U.S. Department of Transportation, 1973), pp. 31–40.

4. B. S. Hetzel, G. A. Ryan, F. McDermott, and E. S. R. Hughes, "Compulsory Blood Alcohol Determinations in Road Crash Casualties—Experience Following Recent Australian Legislation," *Proceedings of the Sixth International Conference on Alcohol, Drugs and Traffic Safety* (Toronto, Ont.: Marketing Services Addiction Research Foundation, 1974).

5. P. M. Moodie, "Mortality and Morbidity in Australian Aboriginal Children," *Medical Journal of Australia 1* (1960), 180.

6. B. S. Hetzel, M. Dobbin, L. Lippmann, and E. Eggleston, *Better Health for Aborigines?* (Brisbane: Queensland Univ. Press, 1974).

7. J. Krupinski and A. Stoller, *The Health of a Metropolis* (Melbourne: Heinemann, 1971).

8. Australian Medical Association, *General Practice and Its Future in Australia,* First Report of the A.M.A. Study Group on Medical Planning (Melbourne: A.M.A., 1972).

9. R. B. Scotton, *Medical Care in Australia—an Economic Diagnosis* (Melbourne: Sun Books, 1974).

10. World Health Organization, *World Health Statistics Annual* (Geneva: WHO, 1974).

11. J. Steinfeld, "Government versus Health 1974," *Annals of Internal Medicine* 81 (1974), 541.

Discussion

Problems and Issues for Consideration

1. How can administrators and policy-makers effectively use epidemiological and health statistics information?

2. What kinds of decisions can be influenced by epidemiological and health statistics information?

3. What are the problems in developing useful epidemiological and health statistics information from both record and survey sources?

4. What are the problems in helping administrators and policy-makers to understand and use this information constructively?

Opening Remarks: John Cassel, M.D.

One of the central problems that has prevented the appropriate use of health statistics for any sort of rational decision-making has been the almost total divorce between those who plan the data system and those who supposedly are going to be using such data for health planning or evaluation. Thus, reporting systems and registers of vital statistics have been planned (and still are) with meticulous attention to questions of standardization of terms, quality of information, record format, coding rules, methods of computerization, retrieval and linkage, not to mention costs and personnel, and when this has all been attended to the keepers of the system find they have a set of data in search of questions. By contrast, administrators, when faced with a problem, look to existing sources of data for help in a solution and are only too often apt to find that much of the available information is either totally irrelevant or at best only marginally helpful. While this is perhaps something of an over-statement, it does, I believe, go a very long way to explain the familiar phenomenon of mountains of data, some analyzed and some not, which regularly gather dust in so many offices across the country. Clearly, the almost reflex scientific response to this problem—more data and perhaps of better quality—is unlikely to provide a solution.

Perhaps the single most important point made by each of the three papers concerned with the problem of application of such data (Mosbech, Holland, and Hetzel) is that they demonstrate that in the three countries described intelligent steps are being taken to rectify this situation. Put in its simplest terms this involves, first, the ability of the administrator, usually in consultation with the epidemiologist or health statistician, to specify in operational terms the nature of the problem facing him. The identification of these problems, for example, financing, management and organization, and content of health services, stems either from the experience of the administrator (such as the familiar set of issues subsumed under the category of scarce resources and multiple demands), or from the results of epidemiological research indicating either that current intervention is of limited or no utility or that new hazards or reasons for the health problems have been identified. Second and of equal importance is the necessity for the administrator to specify the categories of information which would convince him (or his board) of the need for action or which would help make the decision between competing forms of action. This can be an extraordinarily difficult task, both intellectually and organizationally, often requiring a fairly intensive dialogue between administrator and epidemiologist. It is, however, an essential step, as it is on the basis of these decisions that the epidemiologist can decide how much of existing and routine data are useful (or could be made useful) and how much would require new data collection, and if the latter, whether this should be in the form of an ad hoc study or recommended as a subsequent form of routine reporting.

As I indicated, each of the three papers illustrates that, no matter how difficult a task it is, this essential dialogue is 'taking place in the respective countries. The process is more implicit than explicit in Mosbech's paper, but quite explicit in those of Holland and Hetzel. For example, Mosbech indicates the type of information that has led the Danish National Health Service to abandon mass screening for tuberculosis. Presumably, the analysis of these data was undertaken in the face of a recognized potential problem (whether to continue to use personnel and resources for this activity), and the information leading to a decision would have to indicate levels of cost effectiveness. Holland describes a somewhat more complex situation, the hospital facilities needed if St. Thomas's Hospital is to provide total hospital care for the community. Hetzel describes quite explicitly the processes he regards as essential to accomplish this dialogue and reach some form of consensus, including conferences or seminars on neutral ground, and going beyond the professional decision-makers, the involvement of representatives of the community in this process.

In addition to demonstrating that this intelligent planning for and use of epidemiological data can and does take place, the three papers also provide a valuable list of illustrations of the kinds of information that can be provided by epidemiological data. Perhaps a useful classification of these kinds of data would include those that speak to the following six categories:

1. The magnitude and extent of the health problem both in terms of current estimates and trends;

2. The identification of the population groups at highest risk;

3. The elucidation of risk factors, i.e., those environmental and/or behavioral factors that need modification either through the personal health services or through social or political action if the health problem is to be improved;

4. The status of current attempts to alleviate or cope with the problem, both in terms of utilization patterns of existing services and in terms of the impact (effectiveness and efficiency) of the service or procedure;

5. The long-term monitoring of the health consequences of political decisions or changes in the delivery of health services;

6. The surveillance of environmental and behavioral changes to determine their potential health consequences.

Each of these six categories of data and their potential utility has been amply illustrated in these three papers. The extent of chronic uremia and abortions in Denmark and the increased trend in mortality from asthma in young people in Great Britain are illustrations from Mosbech's paper of the first category, the magnitude and extent of the health problem. The appalling infant mortality rate in Australian aborigines (Hetzel) and the poor growth rates in low social class children (Holland) are examples of the identification of populations at high risk. The role of overdose from "Medihalers" in mortality from asthma and PVC (polyvinyl chloride) as a factor in liver cancer (Mosbech) and the importance of cigarette smoking and of respiratory disease in the first year of life for subsequent respiratory disease (Holland) are examples of the identification of risk factors. Holland's studies on early discharge from hospital, Mosbech's and Holland's illustrations of the limitations of screening, and Hetzel's data on automobile injuries and fatalities all illustrate the fourth category of data, the status of current attempts to cope with a problem. Finally, Holland's National Health and Growth Study and Mosbech's comment of the putative role of soft water in cardiovascular mortality are good examples of the potentiality for monitoring the health consequences of political actions and the development of surveillance methods to determine future environmental hazards (such as the introduction of water softeners).

While numerous other examples doubtless could be quoted, these examples, some relatively straightforward and some more complex, are illustrations not of what could be done, but of what is being done by collaboration between well-trained administrators and epidemiologists.

Holland very properly introduces some caveats concerning the difficulties that plague this relationship, including the conflict between the particular and the general and the difference in time scale within which the two groups are working. To these I would add the lack of training or experience on the part of most administrators in specifying their problems in operational terms and identifying the appropriate categories of information needed for their solution, and the inexperience of epidemiologists to determine how much departure from the ideal research design can be tolerated in the face of practical constraints without compromising the validity of the data.

Recognizing these difficulties, however, it behooves us to ask how much of this type of dialogue is going on in the United States in an attempt to solve some of the pressing problems that plague our health service delivery and what are the reasons why this does not occur more extensively. I suspect part of the answer lies in the training of our administrators and epidemiologists. As far as epidemiologists are concerned we have very few training programs which focus on the particular issues involved in applying epidemiological methods to health service issues. Those few that exist have either been phased out or are in danger of such a fate as a result of a series of decisions (and non-decisions) in Washington. But neither for administrators nor for epidemiologists do we have the training opportunities described by Acheson, a central feature of which is the intimate relationship between the theory being presented and the real problems being faced in the field. It is under these conditions that the users of epidemiology can learn these essential skills, which include the ability to delineate problems in operational terms and to learn the rules of evidence—that is, when it is permissible and when not to draw cause and effect conclusions from observational data—which will allow them to collaborate with, but not be at the mercy of, epidemiologists. Similarly, under the conditions described by Acheson, epidemiologists could learn the limitations as well as the potentialities of their discipline and its methods when applied to urgent problems in the field. Perhaps the closest we come to this position in the United States is the Clinical Scholars Program sponsored by the Robert Wood Johnson Foundation. This program, while not intended to produce either health administrators or professional epidemiologists, is designed to educate clinicians in many of the same disciplines mentioned by Acheson to produce medical statesmen of the future. The limited number of such scholars who will be trained, however, will in no way be adequate for the needs of this country, nor could they replace the need for well-trained health administrators and competent epidemiologists capable, to use the words quoted by Acheson, of "accurately measuring the needs of the population both sick and well" and translating these needs into policy and practice.

Summary of General Discussion

1. *Sources of trainees in community medicine and epidemiology in Great Britain.*
The people being trained are basically newly qualified physicians who have completed a clinical internship and who then go to one of the four schools mentioned by Dr. Acheson or to a consortium. These are young physicians whose training parallels very closely the training of surgeons or other specialists, in terms of both salary and time scale. The salary scale is identical, and in the situation that the consortium trains them, they are doing residencies. In universities they go full time but they have to do their residencies as well. At the London School of Hygiene Centre for Extension Training in Community Medicine, there are people who are mature professionals, coming primarily from public health. Some

come from hospital administration, the overseas medical services, and so forth, and are people who have had experience in public health or hospital administration.

2. *Availability of effective health information in Great Britain.*
Because the community physician has no time for detailed and deliberate information-gathering to answer specific questions, information will have to be collected from hospital records, manpower information, treasury information, the matching of costs to diseases, and organized in such a way that this information is retrievable as needed. This is being done in England on a regional basis, instead of on a national basis. The ultimate success of the endeavor depends on clerks and upon physicians. If the physicians are interested, the clerks will do the work. The physicians themselves are only required to enter the diagnosis, while everything else can be done by nontrained workers. However, if the physician is not interested, problems of validity of data inevitably arise, and once this becomes known the results can be invalidated and no one will pay attention to the output. This is the kind of problem referred to by Dr. Hetzel, that of effecting a change in the attitude of the people in a society toward the needs of that society. If the attitude is well developed, and in Great Britain there are regions where it is, systems work quite well. If, on the other hand, a surgeon is at the same time recalcitrant and articulate, it will be a long time before he really cooperates.

3. *Measures to be taken and successes possible in the promotion of the epidemiological perspective in the field of clinical medicine.*
Clear ground rules do not exist in this area, and perhaps the only way to gain the trust, confidence, and cooperation of the clinician is by the epidemiologist's willingness to answer what to him are relatively simple questions which are, however, both interesting and quite difficult from the clinician's point of view. Two examples will illustrate this point. First, at institutions such as St. Thomas's Hospital Medical School, the demands on chemical pathologists are increasing by 10–15 per cent per year, with no concomitant increase in budget. They are, therefore, unable to meet all the requests for tests given to them and so must decide on a system of rationing.

Epidemiologists are able to help these pathologists to decide on ways in which they can screen the requests for tests that would be acceptable to the physicians and surgeons, thereby making the necessary rationing system applicable and at the same time acceptable to those responsible for the delivery of the service. A second example drawn from the St. Thomas's Hospital Medical School concerns outpatient surgery. Six outpatient operating theaters due to open in 1977 are in the process of construction. The epidemiologist can in this instance help the surgeons, administrators, and nurses devise an experiment which will answer their questions and the questions of general practitioners and community nurses in the Area as to how this relatively new system of outpatient operating will function.

4. *Demand for epidemiologists and epidemiological training in the United States.*

In the United States the situation with regard to promotion of the epidemiological perspective appears to have been changing quite drastically over the past five or six years. On the one hand, departments of epidemiology are currently receiving several requests each month from medical schools to provide well-trained epidemiologists. On the other hand, these same departments are receiving in greatly increasing numbers requests from residents in obstetrics, psychiatry, medicine, and pediatrics for training in epidemiology. Further, there are requests coming increasingly from the organized areas of medicine such as the medical societies and organizations and from practitioners to be placed in contact with epidemiologists for help with their ongoing work. The problem from this vantage point, then, is to find and furnish the people, rather than to persuade the clinicians.

IV

EPIDEMIOLOGY,
HEALTH STATISTICS,
AND CONTEMPORARY
HEALTH PROBLEMS

11
W. ESTLIN WATERS, M.D.

THE TEACHING OF EPIDEMIOLOGY AND HEALTH STATISTICS IN A NEW COMMUNITY-ORIENTED MEDICAL SCHOOL

Introduction

The three basic types of discipline in the medical students' curriculum are 1) the preclinical or laboratory sciences; 2) clinical work; and 3) epidemiology and the social sciences. Historically, the first two existed alone and it is comparatively recently that epidemiology and the social sciences became part of the curriculum in most medical schools. Thus medical students have long been taught the importance of the individual as the unit for clinical medicine. They understand, in some detail, about the individual's subdivisions into physiological systems, organs, tissues, cells and even know a little about intracellular structure. But it is only recently that they have had disciplines that have units larger than the individual (populations) as the basis for the discipline. In the United Kingdom the establishment of independent departments of social and preventive medicine, as they were often called, has progressed over the past quarter of a century. In general, as Susser (1) has observed, these departments have pursued their research interests separately from the practitioners of public health (the Medical Officers of Health) and from clinicians. While many departments became centers of academic excellence, the effect of their research on public policy or clinical medicine was sometimes disappointing. In part because of this, there was often a problem of making their teaching appear relevant to medical students. The time allotted in the curriculum was usually very limited.

The report of the Royal Commission on Medical Education 1965–68 (The Todd Report) has had a considerable, but very uneven, effect on medical education in the United Kingdom (2). The Royal Commission recommended in 1967 a new medical school at Southampton. The first intake of students was in October 1971, one year after the school at Nottingham started; it is the only other new medical school in this century in the United Kingdom. The general structure of the medical school and the curriculum have been given by Acheson (3, 4). Three features of the school are important to note here. Firstly, the school is based not only on Southampton with a population of 200,000 but on the whole Wessex region, an area in central southern England with a population of two and a half million. For example, several of the professorial appointments are, in fact, based outside Southampton. Secondly, the curriculum has been planned as a single exercise, with integrated teaching wherever possible. In particular there is no sharp division into preclinical and clinical sections and the students experience a gradually increasing amount of clinical work from their very first term. The third important feature of the Southampton curriculum is that the fourth year (of five) gives each student an opportunity to study one of the wide range of options in depth. With the steady increase in the number of new subjects in the medical curriculum, including such subjects as epidemiology and medical statistics, sociology and psychology, it is increasingly important that each student study one subject in greater detail. Working under the direction of a tutor, a student in his fourth year is permitted to work independently and is provided educational as opposed to vocational training. The Medical Act of 1886 stipulated that, at qualification, a doctor should possess "the knowledge and skill required for the efficient practice of medicine, surgery, and midwifery." However, the Royal Commission on Medical Education (1968) started from the premise that every doctor who wishes to exercise a substantial measure of independent clinical judgment "will be required to have a substantial postgraduate professional training" (5). The Royal Commission continued, "the aim of the . . . course should be to produce not a finished doctor but a broadly educated man who can become a doctor by further training." With the concept that medical education is a continuing process extending right up to retirement, the role of the medical school changes. It is not only what doctors know on the day they qualify that is important, but how equipped they are to continue to learn throughout their professional careers. As the role of the medical school changes, so too should its curriculum. Epidemiology and medical statistics have a very important educational role in this respect.

Why Teach Epidemiology to Medical Students?

Epidemiology is defined in this paper in its broadest sense as the science of the distribution and determinants of disease and disability in human populations, and this is taken here to include the study of the medical needs of society. According to a World Health Organization symposium (6), epidemiological studies have three main purposes:

to guide the development of health services by defining the size and distribution of disease in the community;

to reveal the etiology of disease and hence permit control or modification of the disease;

to provide methods of measuring the effectiveness of medical services.

The aims of teaching epidemiology to medical students are numerous. An important contribution that epidemiology makes is the realization that the standard of health in the community is by no means determined only by the traditional clinical specialities of medicine, surgery, and so forth. "As modern society turns from an almost exclusive interest in the care of individuals who are ill toward an organized effort to preserve the health of a population, it is imperative that all physicians have a grounding in epidemiology" (7). Epidemiology thus gives a medical student an understanding of the interactions between man and environment, of the cause of disease, of the frequency of diseases in populations and of how these frequencies are changing (and perhaps why they are changing). It teaches a critical attitude to both the effectiveness and efficiency of medical care. It gives medical students a broader horizon and greater perspective at the same time as teaching specific epidemiological methods used in studying disease. It is usual to justify the teaching of epidemiology, as with many other subjects, by stating that this is desirable for recruitment into the discipline. However, it is true that many, if not most, of the present generation of epidemiologists were never taught the subject as medical students. The need for epidemiologists, in the future, is likely to continue to increase. It is important to stress the educational role of epidemiology in the curriculum. Consideration of the reasons for teaching epidemiology indicates that every medical student should be exposed to it and that it should not simply be one elective among many others.

With the increasing realization that the maintenance of health in populations is a complex ecological problem there is a growing need for doctors to understand the great importance of preventive medicine and the necessity to organize the delivery of medical care in an efficient way. With an increasing technology these problems will become still more complex. Unless the majority of doctors who are in clinical medicine realize these aspects there is a very real danger that they may take too narrow a view of medicine, to the detriment of the health of those whom they seek to serve. It is essential for all medical students to appreciate these wider aspects of health. A proportion may become involved more directly in the allocation of priorities and medical administration. Although this is a subject for postgraduate study, it is desirable for all doctors to have at least some knowledge of this field because, even as clinicians, they will have to work within the constraints of one of the systems of health care.

Why Teach Medical Statistics to Medical Students?

It is tempting to say that this question has already been answered, at least in the United Kingdom, by Sir Austin Bradford Hill's excellent book *Principles of Medical Statistics* originally published in 1937 and now in its ninth edition (8). However, difficulties still remain. The following is a quotation from the 1965 *Report of the Committee on Social Studies* (9).

Without mathematics and statistics the social sciences as a whole cannot flourish. They are necessary in both the collection and the treatment of data. . . . This need for students to be able to understand statistics and use them intelligently presents a problem. Many opt for the social sciences whose weakness in mathematics deters them from courses in the natural sciences.

Though this was written about the social sciences it applies equally to medicine. Teaching statistics to students can often be combined with epidemiology (10) and in the United Kingdom it frequently is taught by the same departments. Statisticians usually (and rightly) regard statistics in medicine as being relevant to more than epidemiology. It is important, for example, in many of the preclinical sciences. It is true, however, that in most medical schools epidemiology and statistics are closely linked and this symbiosis seems to work well in practice.

The purpose of teaching statistics to medical students has been defined as "to help doctors to think quantitatively and to be able to assess probabilities" (11). Some knowledge of statistics is essential in order to read and understand even the more general medical journals. Statistics, therefore, are one of the important aspects of a medical education. Understanding statistics will enable a doctor to continue to evaluate new ideas and treatments throughout his professional life.

Teaching of Epidemiology and Medical Statistics at Southampton

The Medical School at Southampton has 54 hours of curriculum time for the Epidemiology and Medical Statistics course. The course aims are to demonstrate the scientific validity and medical importance of studies involving groups and populations. It also aims to develop in the medical student, in cooperation with other disciplines, critical attitudes to preventive and therapeutic procedures and to differing methods of organization and delivery of medical care. The main course is in the second term of the second year. In addition, some of the teaching time has been integrated into several of the systems courses (e.g., cardiovascular and respiratory systems courses) during the first and second years. This integrated teaching is usually in the form of symposia with physiologists, clinicians, and pathologists.

Before the Epidemiology and Medical Statistics course there is a course of 24 hours in the very first term entitled "Man, Medicine, and Society." This introduces the student to epidemiology and to the social sciences and demonstrates their relevance to medicine. It also shows the importance of populations and groups as units of study. Following this introductory course there are separate courses in psychology (54 hours) and sociology (54 hours). Epidemiology and medical statistics, psychology and sociology are then examined together in four hours of examination, the Intermediate Part I examination, which is held at the end of the fifth term. This is one of four major examinations and is the only one in the second year.

The main Epidemiology and Medical Statistics Course consists of lectures, statistical practicals, small group seminars and group project work, with the students themselves reporting the findings of their projects to the class. Epidemiological exercises of a modified Terris (12) type are used in small groups. In an effort to show the importance of experimental design, and the danger of acceptance of "views" in clinical medicine without further evidence, an experiment involving beer-tasting has been used (13).

As mentioned above, during the fourth year, students in addition to continuing their clinical work undertake an individual project in consultation with a tutor. This is in effect an "honors type" year, but for all students. In addition a number of courses relevant to nearly all projects are given which cover the design of studies and the collection, handling, and analysis of data. Thus, at the time when students are actually grappling with these problems, their earlier experiences of these subjects are reinforced and extended.

There is not a consensus about when epidemiology and medical statistics should be taught to medical students. It is usually thought that it should be introduced early, before the student becomes too preoccupied with clinical medicine (14). Statistics in particular seems suitable for the first or second year of the medical curriculum as it is also of use in the preclinical sciences. Students at this time have an open and constructively critical mind and are receptive to the broad ecological ideas of epidemiology. The more clinical aspects concerning the epidemiology of particular diseases are rather more difficult to teach at this stage, but the approach should be one of principles rather than of too much detail. Further, if the student learns some clinical medicine at the same time, he will be all the more interested. As most students are particularly interested in clinical medicine it might seem desirable to link the two together, preferably at the bedside or in the community, whenever possible. This method of teaching epidemiology is often time-consuming and in the United Kingdom most epidemiologists in medical schools have moved away from clinical work. At Southampton two of the three epidemiologists have a clinical commitment in a hospital. This is probably useful in getting the subject "accepted" by students and it also allows some of the students to be taught clinical medicine by an epidemiologist. Also at Southampton, there is a very close association with a university general practice of some 5,000 patients. Epidemiologists and university general practitioners share accommodation in the Academic Block at Southampton General Hospital. A temporary health center close by is being replaced by a permanent one, the first in this country to be funded by the University Grants Committee. There is also a close relationship with the Medical Information Unit under Professor Michael Alderson, based twelve miles away at Winchester. This unit is developing methods for monitoring the accuracy and appropriateness of data routinely available in the Health Service. Also in Winchester is Albert Kushlick's Health Care Evaluation Research Team which evaluates services for the mentally handicapped and for the elderly in the Wessex region. Both these groups play an active part in teaching medical students. Finally, it is worth mentioning that several important links are now being established with the Community Medicine specialists since the reorganization of the National Health Service in April 1974. At Southampton Medical School we are therefore attempting, as the Royal Commission on Medical Education (5) recommended we should, "to develop close relations between those working in all the branches of the health services."

Thus, although most of the formal teaching of epidemiology and medical statistics is done in the course of the second year, some of this is reinforced and expanded during the fourth-year projects which all students do.

Resource Materials for Teaching

In each medical school the number of teachers in epidemiology and medical statistics is usually small. This makes contacts with other medical schools highly desirable. Many of the meetings and conferences that academic staff attend are concerned entirely with research topics, but increasingly there is discussion about teaching. At the International Epidemiological Association's Seventh International Scientific Meeting in Brighton, England, in 1974, there was a highly successful and well-attended workshop on teaching methods. International collaboration is important as epidemiology and medical statistics are a new and expanding component in the medical curriculum of most medical schools. Although each country has its particular problems, and epidemiology and medical statistics should be made relevant to these problems, there is much that is common to many countries. The success of the International Epidemiological Association's *Epidemiology: A Guide to Teaching Methods* (14) and its several translations is evidence of this common ground. The limited staff to teach these subjects, and the increasing number of medical students that many schools are taking, makes epidemiological exercises of the type pioneered by Terris (12) very useful. There is also a place for the slide/tape method of learning in epidemiology and medical statistics which has proved so successful at McMaster University. With both these methods a considerable amount of time is required to plan and prepare the material and for this reason international collaboration in such programs should be encouraged. Local modifications of such material will usually be required to make them relevant to students in any particular medical school. Such modifications, however, are usually considerably easier than preparing completely new material. Papers and discussion on teaching methods should continue to be encouraged at both national and international epidemiological meetings so that experience can be passed from one medical school to another. In this way, we can work toward the view of the Goodenough Committee (15) that "the ideas of social medicine must permeate the whole of medical education."

References

1. M. Susser, "Teaching Social Medicine in the United States," *Milbank Memorial Fund Quarterly* 44 (1966), 389.

2. M. D. Warren, and R. M. Acheson, "Training in Community Medicine and Epidemiology in Britain," *International Journal of Epidemiology* 2 (1973), 371.

3. E. D. Acheson, "Medical School at Southampton," *British Medical Journal* 2 (1969), 750.

4. ———, *About Southampton Medical School* (Southampton: Univ. of Southampton, 1974).

5. *Royal Commission on Medical Education, 1965–68, Report,* Cmnd. 3569 (London: Her Majesty's Stationery Office, 1968).

6. WHO Regional Office for Europe, *The Teaching of Epidemiology in Medicine and Public Health: Report on a Symposium* (Copenhagen: World Health Organization, 1968).

7. J. H. Moxley, III, "Epidemiology in Medical Education," *International Journal of Epidemiology* 2 (1973), 367.

8. A. Bradford Hill, *Principles of Medical Statistics,* 9th ed. (London: Lancet, 1971).

9. *Report of the Committee on Social Studies,* Cmnd. 2660 (London: Her Majesty's Stationery Office, 1965).

10. WHO Regional Office for Europe, *Symposium on the Teaching of Statistics to Undergraduate Medical Students in Europe* (Copenhagen: World Health Organization, 1962).

11. Society for Social Medicine, "Evidence Submitted to the Royal Commission on Medical Education," *British Journal of Preventive and Social Medicine* 20 (1966), 153.

12. M. Terris, "The Teaching of Epidemiology to Medical Students," *Archives of Environmental Health* 12 (1966), 801.

13. M. J. Gardner, "An Experiment in Beer-Tasting," *British Journal of Medical Education* 3 (1969), 203.

14. *Epidemiology: A Guide to Teaching Methods*, eds. C. R. Lowe and J. Kostrzewski (Edinburgh and London: Churchill Livingstone, 1973).

15. *Report of the Interdepartmental Committee on Medical Schools* (London: Her Majesty's Stationery Office, 1944).

12
JAN KOSTRZEWSKI, M.D.

TEACHING METHODS IN EPIDEMIOLOGY: EXPERIENCE WITH A GUIDE FOR TEACHERS

Introduction

Modern medicine aspires to learn in detail the structure and function of the human organism from its origin until death, both in health and in disease. On the other hand, it also aims at knowing the factors determining normal or abnormal human development both of a single human being and of the population, and at learning the factors which influence the health of human communities.

The first field of studies involves mainly molecular biology, comprising biochemistry, biophysics, genetics, and immunology as well as other branches of human physiology and pathology, which are the basis for progress in modern diagnostic and therapeutic medicine. The second is based mainly on epidemiology, which deals with factors determining the frequency and distribution of diseases and other health phenomena in human populations. Development of both types of studies has resulted in elaboration of new diagnostic methods, the detection of new drugs and preventive measures, and improvement in therapeutic and prophylactic procedures. Parallel to the development of therapeutic medicine, epidemiology develops consciousness of human needs in the community at large; this, in turn, forces revision of the concepts and organization of the health services. The conventional concept which has concentrated mainly upon clinical medicine and upon the sick person as an individual is not sufficient for all the current health problems associated with contemporary life; it is supplemented by the concept of community medicine which is concerned with the total health problems of the population of a given area (town, district, province, or country as a whole), including those arising from the environment.

Modern Concept of a Comprehensive Health Service System

The concept of the protection of a community's health requires a broad approach to health problems and to the organization of measures for health protection. Besides improvement and further development of curative medicine, that is, organization of medical aid and medical care, more dynamic development of preventive medicine on the one hand, and of rehabilitative medicine on the other hand, is necessary. In this context rehabilitation should be understood as clinical as well as vocational rehabilitation and social readaptation of invalids and the handicapped to viable life in the community.

Proper development of preventive medicine implies, inter alia, creation of proper organization and development of health services responsible for environmental health. The results of studies on environmental health, especially monitoring of environmental pollution and epidemiological surveillance, should be the basis for working out an aggressive program of improvement of the natural environment. This, in turn, should not be adversely influenced by the development of industry and urbanization, or by the use of agricultural chemicals resulting in unnatural modifications of food supplies. This program, once introduced, should be systematically evaluated and modified according to the results of this evaluation. Medical and vocational rehabilitation as well as readaptation to the community of physically or mentally handicapped persons are at present largely in the formative stages of service organization, appropriate for conditions and needs in various countries. The detailed programs and precise concepts of organization of medical and vocational rehabilitation services, social readaptation services, as well as social welfare services are being worked out. The organizational concept of community-oriented comprehensive health service systems embracing preventive, curative, and rehabilitative medicine has been followed by new education programs for physicians, nurses, and social workers. In all this planning, the contribution of epidemiology should be kept in mind.

Elaboration of a comprehensive program for an integrated, community-oriented health service demands an epidemiological approach to definition and quantification of the health and disease problems of the population. This, in turn, requires a fundamental education in epidemiology and health statistics for several groups of people. Evaluation of the health status of the population is indispensable for working out the programs of health protection and assessment of these programs. This cannot be achieved without proper knowledge of epidemiology and health statistics. Without this knowledge it is also impossible to improve the system of health services and to make the system more effective and efficient, nor can cyclic programming or evaluation of the concrete program be carried out.

Need for Epidemiological Education of Physicians and Health Services Administrative Personnel

Epidemiology is the basic discipline for administrators and others concerned with community health services. It is the method used for diagnosis and evaluation of the state of health of the population as well as of the present health needs of the people, and for the estimation of their future needs. Epidemiology is also a valuable tool for evaluation of health service activities. To quote:

In many parts of the world problems facing health services, methods of describing and controlling diseases, and patterns of health care are all changing rapidly. To understand and control these changes requires the widespread use of epidemiological methods and other population-based quantitative techniques, and demands the evaluation of new approaches. There will therefore be an increasing need for specialists in epidemiology and for an appreciation of the value and application of their techniques by the health-care profession as a whole. In the wake of these changing needs and opportunities a new kind of epidemiology is emerging and this must be reflected, in the future, by a different type of training.

Epidemics, despite national and international methods of control, will remain a threat. With rising standards of living, health expectations and investment, there will be increasing public demand for more effective methods of control, and this will require better and faster methods of ascertainment. New diseases will be recognized as the consequence of a combination of new and old environmental exposures. The pattern of existing disease may change in relative frequency and in forms of presentation. The changes will arise from changes in the frequencies and intensities of the multiple factors which are related to these diseases, and from new interactions between the environment, infective and non-infective agents and the genetic structure of the populations concerned. . . . The use of national resources to control disease will need to rest upon strategic decisions supported by more accurate quantitative descriptions of the relationships between these variables, by better measurement and prediction of the effectiveness and efficiency of different intervention techniques and by a greater understanding of the health care system as a whole (1).

International Guide to Teaching Methods in Epidemiology

The adjustment of the health service system to meet the health needs of populations requires fundamental education in epidemiology for each health service worker; it also demands specialists in epidemiology to work in various branches of the health service, especially in administration, preventive medicine, programs in environmental health, and so forth. Epidemiology also has the potential of playing a critical role in the planning and evaluation of health services and can contribute in various ways to health services planning. It enables one to make precise measurements of clearly defined phenomena or to perform experiments which throw light on the effectiveness and efficiency of particular procedures or services which are parts of the whole system. Using epidemiological reasoning it is possible, taking into account past trends together with all the other available relevant data, to predict future health patterns. Epidemiological observations and measurements also make it possible to determine whether implemented plans are leading toward declared objectives (2). The International Epidemiological Association, keeping in mind the increasing needs for education in the principles of epidemiology of all qualified health services workers and for education of specialists in epidemiology, required by the health services in all countries, decided to contribute to this education by preparing a guide to teaching methods in epidemiology.

Epidemiology: A Guide to Teaching Methods (1) should serve all countries, developing as well as developed, and should be applicable to the needs of every system of health care organization, independently of the degree of health service development. In order to make the *Guide* useful in different countries and in different teaching conditions, the International Epidemiological Association invited the collaboration of twenty-six experienced teachers of epidemiology and prominent epidemiologists oriented toward the needs for teaching epidemiology on an international scale from Australia, Czechoslovakia, England and Wales, France, Hungary, India, Israel, Japan, Mexico, Nigeria, Northern Ireland, Poland, Tanzania, the United States, the Union of Soviet Socialist Republics, Venezuela, and from WHO in Geneva. The program for the preparation of the Guide was worked out by two co-editors. One of them teaches epidemiology in Cardiff, Wales, the other one in Warsaw, Poland. In accordance with the plans for preparation of the Guide, each of the twenty-six co-authors prepared an appropriate chapter or its part and presented his teaching program with examples of different forms of teaching in his own setting. Materials developed in this way were used by the editors to prepare a preliminary draft which was then sent to all the authors for comments and suggestions. The next revised version was circulated again to the authors who were subsequently invited by the Polish Academy of Sciences to attend a workshop at Nieborow, Poland for preparation of the final draft of the Guide. Within four days (April 21–24, 1971), the shared effort by individuals from the International Epidemiological Association, the World Health Organization, and the Polish Academy of Sciences resulted in construction of the final draft of the Guide in English.

The Guide was published in 1973, first in Polish, then in English, French, Spanish, Serbo-Croatian, and German. The French edition was purchased for the needs of French-speaking countries by WHO, which also purchased part of the English edition. The Spanish edition was published by the Pan American Health Organization to meet the demands of Spanish-speaking countries. The other editions were published at the expense of the interested countries.

The Guide presents an example of international cooperation by scientists interested in the improvement of the health care of populations all over the world. Completion of this task was possible thanks to the organizational help of the International Epidemiological Association and the World Health Organization, and to the financial support of the Commonwealth Fund of New York, the King Edward's Hospital Fund of London, the Polish Academy of Sciences, and other agencies. Attention should be drawn to the fact that the work of the authors and the editors was donated to the promotion of the health of the world population.

Poland: An Example of Use of the Guide to Teaching Methods in Epidemiology

The National Health Service was introduced in Poland over twenty-five years ago, and as a result of experience and continuous improvement it stands up well to modern demands. It is an integrated system comprising the elements of preventive, curative, and rehabilitative medicine. It also encompasses free health protection and health care for the whole population as well as social welfare for that part of the population in need of help (Figure 12–1). For twenty-five years medical education has been the responsibility of the Ministry of Health. Medical and pharmaceutical faculties were separated from the universities in 1951, and medical schools, called medical academies, were established. There are now ten medical academies under the Ministry of Health and one under the Ministry of Defense. For the last five years the ten medical schools under the Ministry of Health have been functionally connected with the overall health care system.

The link between the medical academies and the health service system is organized on a regional basis (Figure 12–2). Each medical school is linked with two or three provinces. Medical academies are charged with five essential tasks:

to provide new graduates in medicine, dentistry, and pharmacy;

to provide postgraduate training for medical school or other professional graduates in the health services;

to carry out research;

to provide services requiring highly specialized competence;

to oversee the quality of health service activities in their own regions.

Each medical academy has a department of social medicine responsible for pre- and postgraduate teaching of epidemiology in its respective region. Independent of these epidemiology teaching centers, for a quarter century Warsaw has had a viable department of epidemiology in the National Institute of Hygiene. It has been a center for specialty training in epidemology for the whole country.

Using the book *Epidemiology: A Guide to Teaching Methods* (1) the department of epidemiology of the National Institute of Hygiene initiated a seminar for teachers of epidemiology from all the departments of social medicine in Poland in February 1974. As a result of this collaborative effort a program for the teaching of epidemiology was worked out, and the forms and methods of training were accepted and have been introduced in practice. In addition, in June 1974, a seminar was organized for the epidemiologists working at the sanitary epidemiologic stations who were actually involved in teaching epidemiology and in supervision of the two-week practical rotation of fourth-year medical students and for the in-service epidemiology training of regional sanitary-

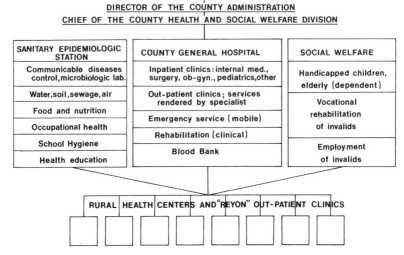

Figure 12–1. Organization of the Polish National Health Service at the County Level.

epidemiologic service workers. In this way the *Guide,* prepared to meet international needs, has been used in practice in Poland.

Future Tasks

The *Guide* may serve as an example of ways in which to continue efforts aimed at the improvement of the methods of epidemiological studies and at popularization of those methods by well-organized international training approaches. Elaboration of valid, simple standard methods for evaluation of the population's health is especially important for planning in the health services and for evaluation of the results of health services planning activities. Different sources of information should be used for evaluation of the population's health; not only commonly used data describing recorded causes of death, incidence of various diseases, injuries, and other health dysfunction, but information concerning the physical and mental development of the population and data about nutrition and other available health indicators. Elaboration of the various health indicators as well as of the principles and methods of collecting, analyzing, and processing of data regarding health conditions of the

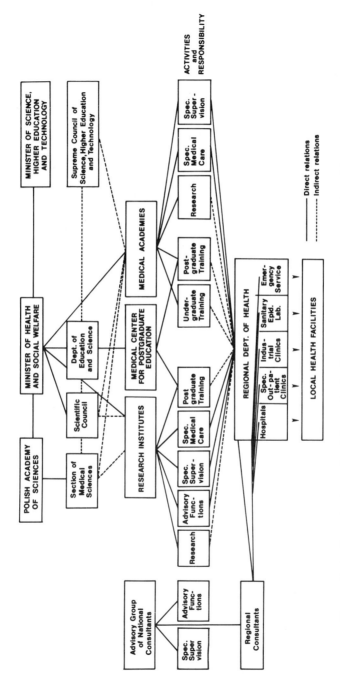

Figure 12–2. Organization of Polish Medical Education Under the Ministry of Health.

population are an important and urgent task. Standardization of these methods will greatly help all countries in their attempts to improve their health service; they will also create a base for international comparisons. This task becomes more urgent as WHO begins its ambitious program of promotion of national health services, while at the same time its Expert Committee on International Classification of Diseases is completing its work on the Ninth Revision of the Classification, enlarged by the new lists of codes that make possible wider and more profound studies on the health state of populations and various influencing factors.

A resolution accepted by the Fifty-fifth Session of the WHO Executive Board in January 1975 asks for expansion of efficient and effective comprehensive health care. It states that large proportions of the population, particularly in rural areas of developing countries have no, or insufficient, access to health services. Therefore, priority should be given to primary health care at the community level as part of a comprehensive health service system including preventive, curative, promotive, and rehabilitative services for the entire populations of countries (3).

References

1. *Epidemiology: A Guide to Teaching Methods,* eds. C. R. Lowe and J. Kostrzewski (Edinburgh and London: Churchill Livingstone, 1973).

2. WHO Regional Office for Europe, *The Application of Epidemiology to the Planning and Evaluation of Health Services* (Copenhagen: World Health Organization, 1973).

3. WHO Executive Board, Fifty-fifth Session, World Health Organization Document EB55.R16 (Geneva: World Health Organization, 1975).

Discussion

Problems and Issues for Consideration

1. Can contemporary problems of medicine, health, and disease be understood without a fundamental education in epidemiology and health statistics?

2. At what point in the continuum of education and professional practice are epidemiology and health statistics most effectively taught and in what settings?

3. What kinds of professionals can most effectively teach the principles, methods, and applications of epidemiology and health statistics?

4. How can we develop through international collaboration resource materials for teaching teachers of epidemiology and health statistics?

Opening Remarks: Robert L. Berg, M.D.

In the case of the average medical student in the United States today, we need to give considerable thought to exactly what amount of epidemiology is needed by any practitioner who will be engaged in the practice of medicine and to consider, from the point of view of economy and efficiency, ways to concentrate our teaching in epidemiology for medical students. Obviously, for those who will be carrying on the work of planning, evaluation, and administration, we have a very different task to perform, but in the case of the prospective health practitioner it is becoming increasingly important to identify that core of epidemiological and statistical understanding which every practitioner needs. The importance of effectively accomplishing this task is emphasized by recent attitudinal changes among United States medical students. In the last ten years there has been a definite shift among medical students away from interest in the community. This is perhaps a reflection of the way they are chosen, of the extraordinary increase in competitiveness for openings in medical schools as the number of people applying for entrance has almost doubled in the last ten years. It is also related to the fact that they want to practice along the lines of the one-to-one doctor-patient relationship of practitioners of the past who serve as their present-day models. This change in attitude among medical students has come on rather rapidly, and, whether or not it is happening elsewhere in the world, we might do well to attend to those areas of good medical practice here that require knowledge of epidemiology and biostatistics and learn ways to deal with them effectively.

Every practitioner must understand the setting in which disease and health care behavior occurs, and those demographic, occupational, social, and community aspects that define how people tend to get health care and how they tend to get diseases. He should be able to identify the risks to which patients are subject, the characteristics which define such risks, that he may have at least an understanding of the strategy of effectiveness of medical therapy. Perhaps every physician, before he goes into practice, should participate in a clinical trial simply to know how extraordinarily difficult it is.

In addition to some of these basic epidemiological ideas, he should have a knowledge of "optimization," how he spends his time and uses the resources available to him; further, in this respect, he needs to go beyond epidemiology to various economic models to which we should bind our epidemiologic teaching in terms of the optimal allocation of resources. The practitioner should know something about evaluation in terms of the processes or outcomes of care, something about sampling, observer error, and standardization. In fact, perhaps instead of a course in epidemiology we should give a course in health care into which the epidemiological methods and skills are woven inextricably so that he will understand how they are used, and why he needs these skills to be an effective practitioner. In my view, such an approach is our only chance at capturing this particular generation of medical students. I think it would be desirable to present epidemiology in a primary care setting, especially with care given to defined populations. At Rochester we have found that our greatest success lies in putting first-year students into the family medicine programs and into prepaid group practices where the notion of a defined population, or of a population for whom one has accepted care, is well articulated. A widespread student attitude, epidemiologically informed through looking into efficacy and effectiveness in a large number of clinical trials, will perhaps ultimately help create in every health care delivery system a climate of curiosity, humility, and uncertainty as to how things work or do not work.

The attitude that the practitioner cannot do research is widespread. The emergence of health care research creates a situation in which every practitioner can, in fact, be involved in an exciting climate of research and studies that rotate around his everyday life. Furthermore, the emergence of group practices and Health Maintenance Organizations provides an excellent setting in which a standard of excellence can be determined and laid out. Unless we make the epidemiological and biostatistical disciplines very relevant to what every medical student knows he will be doing, I fear that we will have little success with this particular generation of practitioners in the United States, whose preoccupation lies increasingly with the individual practice of medicine and the individual patient.

Summary of General Discussion

1. *Problems involved in teaching epidemiology in a clinical setting.*
There is a great difficulty in being both an effective epidemiologist and a strong clinician. When visiting the wards, the house staff and medical staff want to see a clinician able to define the intricacies of what they are observing; the training and experience underlying that ability take many years of study. Unfortunately, the clinician-in-training generally receives no exposure to epidemiological ideas during this time, not even the small amount that might enable him to ask the proper questions of the patient so that he could place the patient's problem in a broader perspective. In addition, the student needs to be exposed to a model teacher who is asking such questions. Possibly the most effective site for this type of training is in a group or family practice setting. The University of Maryland School of Medicine has a required rotation, and during one six-week rotation the medical students, in groups of about sixteen, are required to do two half-days in epidemiology. Those days are given over to discussions bearing on the justification of the treatments that

they are using in ambulatory care. This is the most popular course in that part of the senior year and the only one that the students have asked to have extended in their curriculum.

2. *Differences between teaching medical students in Europe and in the United States.*

It has been pointed out that the entire medical education is conducted on a university level starting after secondary school in most European countries, whereas in the United States most students have already finished their undergraduate education where the quantitative disciplines are poorly represented, and the task of redirecting the fuzzy thinking patterns that have developed and are permitted to exist is not easy, particularly when most of the faculty think in similarly nonquantitative and undisciplined manners.

It was also indicated, however, that the basic difficulty both in the United States and abroad is to acquaint the medical student, at whatever level, with the relevance of what one is trying to do. If he can be shown that what he is learning is relevant, the medical student will listen. During periods of social turmoil, he is interested in society and that is the field of relevance. During periods of acquiescence, he is much more interested in the patient and what goes on in the bed, and in that case, he must be interested by working on that basis.

13
LOUIS M. F. MASSÉ, M.D.

EPIDEMIOLOGY
AND CONTEMPORARY
HEALTH PROBLEMS

Introduction

This paper will briefly consider the uses of epidemiology and health statistics in the solution of *contemporary* health problems, as opposed to *categorical* health problems, that is, those health problems arising from one specific disease, or from exposure to one specific hazard. Contemporary health problems are likely to be combinations of several categorical health problems acting in a complex way on a specific group of persons identified by some similarities in the way these shared problems aggregate—for example, large families with low income, handicapped persons, the unemployed, the aged, and so forth. When dealing with these contemporary health problems, it is important to keep in mind the socioeconomic differences existing between four different types of countries, and the health implications of these differences:

developing countries without natural resources;

developing countries with natural resources;

industrialized countries with free market health organizations;

industrialized countries with nationalized health organizations.

From the standpoint of the epidemiologist or health statistician, it is important to stress the distinction between three main approaches to epidemiology and health problems:

descriptive epidemiology;

analytic epidemiology;

comprehensive epidemiology.

Contemporary Health Problems with Special Emphasis on Manifestational Entities

Descriptive epidemiology deals essentially with disease manifestations and the spread of disease in the community. It typically addresses the characteristics of time, place, and persons. Descriptive epidemiology is sometimes roughly referred to as the traditional "public health" use of epidemiology. Analytical research is oriented toward understanding causation, that is, toward finding the agent responsible for the disease entity. So-called "retrospective studies" are the most common initial investigative studies. A better expression would be "studies by anamnesis," the word anamnesis having the advantage of being more specific than the word retrospective and of being in current use in most continental languages; the word retrospective is equivocal even among epidemiologists, and is even more equivocal when epidemiologists deal with economists. Although the study of disease entities is the oldest and still the most common application of epidemiology, there is a rapid change in strategies used for this purpose. Disease entities are not the same as they were a century ago or even ten years ago; even if "disease" did not change, public expectations of health have changed to the extent that the spectrum of disease described in the files of wards, outpatient clinics, or private practitioners must change over time.

Problems in defining conditions at death. The main causes of death for which an epidemiologist or a health statistician had to watch carefully in the past were those against which some sort of quick intervention was possible or urgently needed for the benefit or the protection of the whole group, such as communicable diseases, accidents, or malnutrition. In many industrialized countries, where preventive or curative interventions were usually (although not systematically) successful against these causes of death, most of the deaths now occur after retirement age and are the result of a combination of many concurrent conditions, some of which are difficult to attribute to a specific traditional diagnosis. Simply accounting for causes of death, a major basis for epidemiological activity in the past, is no longer sufficient; more than routine plotting of facts in the appropriate columns of a table and computation of relative frequencies or rates is needed. Combinations of conditions leading to death must be identified and measured in very complex ways, using detailed information about every biological change involved in the terminal process. These data need to be treated by several different types of multivariate procedures, with comparison of the results derived from the various methods leading to selection of the best one for treatment of the data.

Results are sometimes expressed in terms of *risk factors,* the word factor having been borrowed from mathematics. Although the word factor is correct when used alone, the expression "risk factor" is incorrect, because it carries a causal connotation and any causal connotation should be systematically avoided until some proof is given, by an appropriate device, experiment, or randomized control procedure, that a causal relationship really does exist. *Risk indicators,* or *risk markers,* are better expressions to describe these findings. Once demonstrated by an appropriate analysis, these risk markers might help to determine adequate preventive actions, the efficacy, effectiveness, and efficiency of which should be constantly evaluated.

Similar comments apply to the control of perinatal causes of death, a combination of stillbirths and deaths during the first week of life; aside from the needed prevention of delivery accidents by adequate technical facilities in any maternity hospital, it may be necessary to collect more complete information on all the facts of life surrounding mating and pregnancy. Collection of data would require the "symnesis" of genealogies and hospital experiences of both parents in the way suggested below for the Province of Quebec in Canada.

Growing need for a premorbidity appraisal. Morbidity measurement is no longer exclusively the quantitative appraisal of disease patterns; individuals, families and, for other reasons, employers, consider that disease results from accidental defects in health protection or promotion, and that they are entitled to "predisease" protection. As a result, in many countries there is increasing use and demand for private or public medical "checkup" or "screening" systems. A simpleminded computation shows that for a country like France, if every citizen were to request all the "checkups" he is entitled to, according to a law voted in 1946 and very fortunately never systematically enforced so far, a sizable proportion of the public health budget would go into these activities alone. But the existing procedures for these checkups are not adapted to their goals; most of them are still derived from techniques for examinations performed on sick patients; very little is known about their efficacy in forecasting individual risk for apparently healthy subjects, or in guiding the prescription of preventive measures. Before any measurement of efficacy is possible, a descriptive approach by multivariate analysis should yield a classification of minor biological changes, subsymptoms, small deviations of healthy behavior, and any significant groupings of these.

Then, on the basis of these descriptive findings, the measurement of their efficacy as risk markers would require a systematic catamnesis, that is, "follow-up," of subjects to measure subsequent experiences. While these studies take place, many changes will occur in the way such examinations are routinely performed or recorded, making catamnestic comparisons questionable. This technical drift must be considered in making any appraisal.

Enlarged scope of disability. Disability, although essentially liable to persistence, is more difficult to quantify than one would expect. Some disabled persons tend to hide and to avoid contact with those officially in charge of helping them, while others tend to overemphasize their problems if they expect some return or reward.

If physical disability is difficult to measure, more difficult still to define and evaluate is psychological disability. Measurement of I.Q. remains a very controversial activity and emotional disturbances are seen very differently by specialists according to their school of thought. Disability of a psychological nature tends to be communicable; in urban settings, where family ties are loose, it tends to evolve toward drug abuse or violence, thus creating more disturbances. The facts to be recorded and analyzed in this area are more complex than biological data and tend to generate less objective measurements. Further, the standards of deviation acceptance by the community sometimes change rapidly, making any analysis of trends questionable. It is difficult to set up formal limits to the concept of health disability. Social disability is another field that should be covered by the epidemiologist, both for its direct implications and for its indirect consequences on physical or mental health and/or unemployment, hierarchical pressure, and limitations of freedom.

Contemporary Health Problems with Special Emphasis on Exposure to Risk

Analytic epidemiology deals essentially with differences in level of exposure to risk agents. Analytical research is aimed at research of consequences, with the help of the so-called "prospective studies." A more apt expression would be "studies by catamnesis," the word catamnesis having the advantage of being more specific than the word prospective, and having the added advantage of already existing in most of the European continental languages as a medical term with a specific meaning. Analytic epidemiology is sometimes referred to as, roughly, the present "social medicine" level of epidemiology. Exposure to an "environment" might include in some cases exposure to a systematic health procedure, for example, immunization, therapy, and so forth, and, in that particular case, one of the goals of analytic epidemiology will be to study the efficacy of this procedure and, in part, its effectiveness.

Environmental problems are well known to the public; we should, however, remember that they are not restricted to pollution. The main facts for consideration can be classified under the headings congenital, familial, physical, biological, psychological, and socioeconomic environments. Three main subchapters, however, are more usually considered:

maternal and child health;

environmental health;

occupational health.

Maternal and child health. Maternal and child health constitute traditional health problems. Reproductive and pregnancy conditions, physiological or psychological, external factors involved in the growth and development of children, poverty, drug and alcohol problems in the way they affect family life, fertility control, family dietary practices and their determinants, are classic environmental problems involving maternal and familial environments. Present concern is oriented more toward the effect on family structure of migration from rural to urban conditions and toward the consequences of the population explosion on family life in developing countries.

Environmental health. Epidemiologists and health statisticians try to set up the methods for assessment of risk and the evaluation of environmental policies and management. These studies should cover all the sources of environmental pollution:

air (chemical, physical behavior of air and air contaminants);

water (water chemistry, including the classic problem of softness/ hardness of water, water bacteriology and virology, efficiency of water handling and treatment, and of water resources planning, conservation and management, limnology and oceanography);

ionizing radiations (efficacy of radiation protection and interactions with the biological environment);

food, housing, waste disposal, insects, rodents, accidents, heat, light, and noises, and so forth.

Occupational health. Although very important, occupational health has not received enough attention from epidemiologists in many countries. Not only do studies on occupational hazards need to receive more attention and financial support but the efficacy of present programs for the protection and conservation of the working population should be studied, including accident control, occupational health education and, especially for young workers, family health education, including family planning and nutritional health education.

Comprehensive Approach to Contemporary Health Problems

Comprehensive epidemiology deals essentially with health problems derived from complex situations in social life. It uses the tools of demography, operational research, and engineering information systems.

Demography and contemporary health problems. The word demography coined one hundred and twenty years ago, entered the lexicon of the epidemiologist only about fifteen years ago. Before then two expressions were used in the English-speaking countries to cover very nearly the same field of interest: "population studies" and "vital statistics." The fact that the word demography is now largely accepted is considered the consequence of two major factors: first, the growing importance of demographic facts as a result of the long-lasting population explosion in developing countries; and second, in a few European countries, the fact that demography has been a part of the secondary school curriculum for the last twenty years, so that now most of the junior staff of every organization or agency has some background in the field. One can hope that one day the study of epidemiological principles will also become a part of the secondary curriculum so that this particular line of thought will be more readily accepted and even encouraged by nonmedical leaders of the community.

Population data have always been routinely used as a basis for statistical analysis in any epidemiological investigation. Population data were essentially used to provide denominator data for rates and other ratios; more detailed population data by sex, age, and socioeconomic conditions would help to standardize these rates or to identify fractions of populations that are homogeneous as regards the risk of acquiring the condition under study. But population data are now equally used to detect new distributions of the population structure and to draw attention, for instance, to the importance of maternal and child health epidemiology in developing countries (60–70 per cent of the population) or to the importance of geriatrics in industrialized countries (10–15 per cent of the population). Overemphasis of these two major concerns of modern epidemiology has led to at least one objectionable side effect: studies on occupational epidemiology do not attract enough attention and financial support in many countries. Workers themselves seem to show less interest than do those whom they help and support with the products of their work. The only exception to this lack of interest in occupational health is a new interest in the changes occurring in the population structure of women who work in urban areas. In rural areas, whether or not a woman works has little effect on family life, since her work usually takes place within a short distance of the dwelling unit. On the other hand, in urban areas, the consequences of work for women on family life are very important, and analysis of demographic data concerning the changes in the structure of employment can be of great importance as a basis for the epidemiological investigation of exposure of children to new traumatic, nutritional, or psychological hazards, and the services needed to prevent them. Other population studies are related to the demographic structure of all the health professions; medical demography is now a very important tool of health management systems.

The old demographic concept of optimum population, although very popular at one time, has been forsaken during the last thirty years for lack of good criteria on which to base judgments of what is best. But with the present increasing use of epidemiology, it is now possible to express the concept of optimum population in terms of community medicine: the optimum population is that size and structure of a population that makes it possible for a country to organize its health services so that instead of concentrating only on the prevention of disease, the promotion of health within a safe and happy environment can be made available, without exception, to all present human beings and their offspring.

As regards vital statistics, the main concern of the epidemiologists and health statisticians was traditionally aimed at the study of mortality. Today more emphasis is placed on natality and fertility, but to a large extent the field of fertility is no longer studied under the label of demography. Studies made for the benefit of the epidemiologist interested in maternal and child health are given different names in different countries. Some will accept the idea of undertaking a study of the fertility components associated with a happy family life, rather than dealing with the consequences of a population explosion with the objective of population control.

Operational research and contemporary health problems. The definition of the expression "operational research" is different in every country; it is hoped that the following remarks will not contribute to the confusion.

Health care systems can be divided into subsystems, some of which are health information systems; these health information systems are subdivided into two categories: information systems and engineering information systems. *Information systems* comprise one of the tools of operational research. Systems analysis of health problems might be based on various approaches: mathematical models; production functions (benefits and costs); optimization; marginal analysis; linear or nonlinear and dynamic programming; Markov processes; stochastic programming. These information systems should deal not only with the measurement of contemporary health problems per se but also with the measurement of the development of health manpower, of the actions promoting environmental health, of the strengthening of health services, of the use of health planning, of the implementation and results of the management of health services and institutions.

Plans for health services need to avoid the usual danger of health planning, that is, attacking diseases or exposures to risk, or other health problems one by one. Although a comprehensive approach to health care systems is still a new goal very rarely reached in practice, the future of epidemiology and health statistics lies in dealing with a great number of problems by an integrated approach. In order to achieve this multidimensional goal, health information systems should gather appropriate amounts of usable data concerning health, the environment, health services, and health management. The tool for this data handling is the engineering information system.

Engineering information systems and contemporary health problems. An increasingly important area of advance in epidemiology is the development of medical record linkage. So impressive are the results of this that both public interest and public concern have increased. There is a fear that some breach of confidentiality might result from use or abuse of information derived from medical record linkage studies. A small part of this concern may be founded on experience, but a great part is tied up with the fact that the expression "medical record linkage" has been too well coined and says too much. The two words "record" and "linkage" have an indirect connotation of surveillance and spying. (The word "symnesis" would be less obvious.) The achievements of these methods are too well known to need mention, and the results are far too numerous to list here. One example, not yet implemented but with some very specific features, will be described.

In the Province of Quebec, Canada, christenings, marriages, and burials have been carefully recorded by Catholic priests for more than three hundred years. Although this has also been the case in many other countries, Quebec is probably the only area where these records have not been destroyed by war or other circumstances. Most of these records were kept in duplicate, one in the parish district and the other in the local judicial center. Genealogies of the majority of the French Canadian population can thus be established since immigration from Europe and data from these records are currently used by some private firms for establishing genealogies. Research workers from the University of Montreal started years ago to gather microfilm copies of the early records, and, more recently, a computer data bank was set up. A cross check with successive censuses is thereby possible; the first one dates back to 1667. In Quebec, as well as in the whole of Canada, all patients admitted to hospitals, private or public, are covered by a government insurance plan. A hospital discharge abstract and claims form is sent to the government for reimbursement. These forms, gathered and computerized centrally, include details of admission, discharge, length of stay, diagnosis, prescriptions, surgery and responsible physician, and so forth. One day, through a device of individual identification, these two sets of data could be linked together. Since the population of Quebec is relatively small, this linkage is still feasible. Such a system would be beneficial for comprehensive epidemiology in two ways: first, in any study requiring information on hospital admission and on vital events, it would be possible to process all the data together making analysis more interesting; second, genealogies of patients admitted for a genetic condition could be studied to find out, for instance, their common ancestor, if any. From this one could identify descendants and analyze and compare their morbidity patterns; in fact, a familial component might be studied. With such material available, the limiting factor would not be the amount of health data, but rather the lack of financial resources and of trained epidemiologists.

14

ADETOKUNBO O. LUCAS, M.D.

EPIDEMIOLOGY
AND HEALTH STATISTICS
IN THE CONTROL
OF COMMUNICABLE DISEASES

Epidemiology as a science owes its reputation primarily to its successful application in the control of communicable diseases, although it has subsequently proved of value in the study of chronic noninfectious diseases and in the planning and evaluation of health services. With the successful control of some of the major epidemic diseases, it is tempting to think that the problem of communicable diseases has been solved. The availability of antibiotics and other antimicrobial agents has also tended to foster the view that the epidemiological approach no longer deserves emphasis, since effective chemotherapy can always be applied in broad spectrum, blunderbuss fashion to deal with these infections. There is abundant evidence, however, that even though a number of communicable diseases have come under successful control, there is the persistent menace of unsolved problems. Thus, although a number of bacterial infections have declined in frequency, viral infections of the respiratory tract, especially in children, remain important causes of morbidity. In many countries various factors, biological and behavioral, have combined to aggravate the problem of gonorrhea and nonspecific urethritis. It is also important to consider the international dimension of the problem; with the increased pace and volume of international travel, most communicable diseases can be brought to the doorstep of any country from the most distant lands (1).

All these facts indicate the need for continued vigilance for communicable diseases and the continuing application of proven epidemiological techniques in programs for the control of these infections. In this presentation, I will review briefly some of the uses of epidemiology and health statistics in the control of communicable diseases. Apart from the classical traditional techniques of observational and experimental epidemiology, some of the growing areas in the epidemiology of communicable diseases, particularly the new developments in theoretical epidemiology, the use of mathematical models and computer simulation will be examined.

Health Statistics

Analysis of vital statistics, especially births and deaths, can provide basic information about the health of the community. Additional information is derived from notifications of specific diseases. These routinely collected data can be analyzed with regard to the common causes of sickness and death, their distribution by *person, place,* and *time.* Such simple epidemiological analysis provides valuable information about the common causes of sickness and death in the population. It provides simple answers to the three basic epidemiological questions:

Who? Which groups of persons are most seriously affected and which groups are spared?

Where? What is the geographical distribution of the problems?

When? What are the time relationships—peak periods, seasonal variations, time trends, and so forth?

The epidemiologist brings to this analysis the strict discipline of his science with particular reference to:

definitions of variables, using objective criteria as far as possible;

identification and elimination of sources of error in observation, recording, and interpretation, and the measurement of such errors;

validation of the measurements used to determine to what extent the instruments actually measure what the epidemiologist set out to measure; and careful editing and evaluation of the data to ensure that appropriate weight is given to the available evidence.

Routine collection of health statistics, births, deaths, and sickness data provides useful baseline information for the epidemiologist with regard to the relative importance of the major communicable diseases.

Special Investigations

Epidemiological investigations may be promoted by the outbreak of acute infections as, for example, an epidemic of diarrhea and vomiting in an institution. In this type of fire-fighting operation, the epidemiologist attempts to identify and eliminate the source of infection, to protect all those who are at risk, and to take measures to prevent the recurrence of such outbreaks. Special surveys are also carried out to provide information which is complementary to that derived from clinical sources. Such additional information helps to complete the picture by providing information about subclinical and inapparent infections. Applied microbiology and immunology play an important role in epidemiological surveys of infectious diseases, but other methods, for example, routine radiography of the chest, may provide valuable information. Microbiological examination of sputum, urine, feces, skin, and throat can provide information about the prevalence of mild infections and of the carrier state. Carriers, that is, persons who excrete the infective agents of a specific disease without showing clinical signs of infection, play an important role in some infections, for instance, typhoid or cerebro-spinal meningitis:

The *number* of carriers may far exceed the number of clinically apparent cases;

The *duration* of the carrier state may exceed the duration of acute infections; the carrier thus constitutes a danger over a much longer period and may be responsible for the maintenance of the infection within the community in the interepidemic period;

The *activities* of the carrier are not restricted. He does not feel ill; neither he nor his contact is aware that he constitutes a danger. He is thereby exposed to many more contacts than the acutely ill patient.

A variety of immunological tests are used in epidemiological investigations, for example, tuberculin tests. Skin tests which are based on allergic reactions may indicate current infection or previous exposure to specific infections. The theoretical basis for the use of serology in the epidemiological investigation of communicable diseases is simple and quite familiar. Current and recent acute infections may be diagnosed by the characteristic pattern of changes in the serum levels of specific antibodies. Latent infections may be detected by positive serological tests and the antibody components which persist for long periods provide virtually permanent records of previous exposure to various infective agents. Serology is therefore used in the diagnosis of acute infections; it provides more precise identification of the infective agent than can be achieved by clinical methods alone. Subclinical infections can also be detected, thereby widening the scope of epidemiology beyond the limited spectrum of overt disease. Apart from its use in limiting acute epidemics, serological epidemiology has proved valuable in identifying the major public health problems in an area, thereby providing rational guidance for the planning, implementation, assessment, and evaluation of programs for the control of communicable diseases. The pattern of infection in the community may be determined from the examination of sera from representative samples of the population. The frequency and distribution of the infection and level of immunity can be mapped out in terms of such variables as age, sex, geographic location, and socioeconomic factors. After thus outlining the serological profile of the community, the situation can be monitored over the years by the use of repeated surveys or by long-term longitudinal studies. One can thereby detect fluctuations in the level of infection within the community, whether these fluctuations have occurred spontaneously or in response to control programs. Serological surveys have been usefully applied in the planning and assessment of immunization programs against such infections as poliomyelitis and measles. The precampaign serological surveys indicate the susceptible groups within the population and the postimmunization studies provide objective assessment of the success of the program by showing what proportion of the susceptible groups remain unprotected. Such evaluation of measles immunization programs has drawn attention to the fact that this procedure gives relatively poor protection to children who are vaccinated under one year old (2). Serology can also be used to evaluate programs which have been based on mass chemotherapy and environmental control measures directed, for example, at endemic treponematoses and malaria; the residual foci of infection can be indicated and the recrudescence of transmission can be detected by the use of appropriate serological tests. Recent technical developments for collecting, preserving, transporting, storing and processing sera have made it possible to conduct serological surveys even in the most remote areas. In this way, the services of well-equipped reference laboratories, both national and international, and the skill of highly trained technical staff can be made available to remote small rural communities. Mass serological surveys are often planned to include the study of several diseases that are of interest in a particular area; unused portions of sera provide material for conducting exploratory studies on other conditions, infective, hematological and genetic, which are not the primary interest of the study.

Surveillance

During the past twenty years, epidemiologists have developed a new approach to the control of communicable diseases (3, 4). One defect of the traditional system had been the compartmentalization of relevant information. Thus, while the health authorities normally had access to certain "health statistics," other pertinent data were collected and retained by hospital authorities, veterinarians, pharmacists, and laboratory institutes.

The modern concept of surveillance implies the exercise of continuous scrutiny of and watchfulness over the distribution and spread of infections and factors related thereto, of sufficient accuracy and completeness to be pertinent to effective control. Three main steps are involved in the process of surveillance:

the systematic collection of pertinent data;

the orderly consolidation and evaluation of these data; and

the prompt dissemination of the results to those who need to know, particularly those who are in a position to take action.

Surveillance of communicable disease is used for the recognition of acute problems, for example, the outbreak of an epidemic disease, the aim being to confine it to the smallest possible area in the shortest possible time. The technique is also useful for the broad assessment of specific problems in a particular community or country, and for the establishment of priorities; for discerning long-term trends and epidemiological patterns; for providing the scientific basis for ascertaining the advisability and extent of mass vaccination and assessing its effectiveness; and for the early recognition of changes in disease patterns and a prompt adjustment of control measures. Pertinent data may be derived from the following sources:

mortality registration;

morbidity reporting;

epidemic reporting;

laboratory investigations;

individual case investigations;

epidemic field investigations;

epidemiological surveys;

animal reservoir and vector distributions;

biologics and drug utilization;

demographic and environmental data.

It is necessary to set up mechanisms by which pertinent epidemiological data are brought together, where they can be evaluated, correlated, and interpreted by competent epidemiologists, thereby providing the logical basis for effective action. The need for international collaboration in the control of communicable disease has been long recognized. As a further development of the International Sanitary Regulations, the new trend is to use surveillance techniques on an international level. The smallpox eradication program represents one of the most successful outcomes of this approach. The World Health Organization is playing a central role in these international programs.

Mathematical Models and Computer Simulation

Considerable progress has been made in recent years in evolving mathematical theories of epidemics, and a number of mathematical models have proved of practical value in the field (5). Mathematical models can be used to simulate epidemic processes and thereby provide a scientific basis for predicting the expected outcomes of various types of preventive measures. This is particularly valuable in making decisions as to the cheapest and most effective way of tackling a particular situation. Thus mathematical models assist in cost-effectiveness and cost-benefit analyses. In particular situations, they can provide guidance as to the relative values of sanitation and immunization in the control of a feco-oral infection like typhoid or cholera (6). These complex mathematical calculations involving several variables have been rendered manageable by the use of electronic computers.

Conclusion

Epidemiology provides the logical scientific basis for the control of communicable diseases. It defines the distribution of the disease within the community and helps identify the determinant factors. Epidemiological surveillance provides an integrated information system which can keep these diseases under continuous scrutiny, thereby providing a valid basis for making decisions about the most appropriate interventions required to control these diseases. It also assists in the evaluation of the response to such interventions.

References

1. R. G. A. Sutton, "An Outbreak of Cholera in Australia Due to Food Served in Flight on an International Aircraft," *Cambridge Journal of Hygiene* 72 (1974), 441–45.

2. C. C. Linnemann, Jr., "Measles Vaccine: Immunity, Reinfection and Revaccination," *American Journal of Epidemiology* 97 (1973), 365–71.

3. A. D. Langmuir, "The Surveillance of Diseases of National Importance," *New England Journal of Medicine* 268 (1963), 182–92.

4. K. Raska, "National and International Surveillance of Communicable Diseases," *WHO Chronicle* 20 (1966), 315–21.

5. N. T. J. Bailey, *The Mathematical Theory of Epidemics* (London: C. Griffin & Co., 1957).

6. B. Cvjetanović, K. Uemura, B. Grab, and T. Sundaresan, "Use of Mathematical Models in the Evaluation of the Effectiveness of Preventive Measures Against Some Infectious Diseases," in *Uses of Epidemiology in Planning Health Services,* Proceedings of the Sixth International Scientific Meeting of the International Epidemiological Association, ed. A. M. Davies (Belgrade: Savremena Administracija, 1973), Vol. II, pp. 913–933.

Discussion

Problems and Issues for Consideration

1. How can epidemiology and health statistics be used to define the extent and nature of health problems, the populations at greatest risk of experiencing them, and to describe the change in patterns of problems and of populations?

2. How can epidemiology and health statistics be used to identify the times, places, and groups for maximum intervention?

3. How can epidemiology and health statistics be used to assist politicians, administrators, and planners in setting priorities and allocating resources?

4. How can epidemiology and health statistics be used to evaluate the efficacy, effectiveness, and efficiency of health care?

Remarks: J. Thomas Grayston, M.D.

One of the important messages for me from the papers of Professors Lucas and Massé is that we have come a long way toward a general

understanding and agreement concerning the definition of epidemiology. Some of the repetitiousness of today's presentations indicates that
epidemiological techniques are being applied widely and with a common vocabulary of understanding to a variety of health problems, including health care delivery.

While the papers presented here do not mean to imply acceptance of
the one-to-one patient-physician model as the only way to deliver
health services, little attention has been paid to defining an optimal
framework for delivery of economical and effective health care. This
question is very important to us today and is susceptible, at least in
part, to study by epidemiological techniques. One major problem confronting us at present is the proper mix of health professionals in various
parts of the delivery system. Without such information we are trying to
face the manpower problems of how many more doctors, nurses, and
other health professionals are needed. It is a very pressing problem and
one susceptible to the use of epidemiological techniques, not so much
to answer the questions, for they go beyond epidemiological data into
the political arena, but to provide hard data for informed decisions concerning health manpower needs.

An issue illustrative of the utility of epidemiological data in confronting health manpower problems occurred recently in Washington State,
where the local optometrists association, supported by their national
group, have requested establishment of a College of Optometry at the
University of Washington. It was clear that simple epidemiological techniques could provide very useful data in the study of whether this was
something that needed to be done. Both numerator (optometrists in
practice) and denominator (population data from the state) were looked
at from the point of view of both rural and urban distributions, along
with national comparative data. These data were useful in arriving at a
conclusion about the need for such a school in our state, which along
with resources and other factors within the university allowed a position to be taken. The matter is in the political arena now, still unre-
solved, but provided with some reasonable data to address to the
problem.

One of the difficulties in bringing about a more rational structuring
of manpower in the health care delivery system is the "professionalism"
of the various health professional groups. Two experiences emphasize
the universality of this problem. First, there exists in Washington state a
Board of Licensure for nurses, derived from a new, more liberal Nurse
Practice Act. This group has established the definition of a new type of
specialized nurse practitioner, and one of the qualifications for this
status is a Master's Degree in Nursing. Second, there is at present a
group of University of Washington faculty looking into the appropriate-

ness of clinical pharmacy instruction in our university hospital. They are studying some of the programs elsewhere in the country in their search for ideas. It was reported to them by the dean of a school of pharmacy that he felt unequivocally that no more pharmacists should be graduated without the Doctor of Pharmacy degree. The point of these two illustrations is that, while numerous statements have been presented about frustrations in dealing with the professionalism of physicians and dentists and in getting them to understand some of the things that are obvious to epidemiologists about how manpower could be more efficiently deployed, other health professionals are attempting through the educational system to enhance their status and to add rigidity to the system. Perhaps the idea of the epidemiologist standing with a strong administrator and looking at the total problem has some advantage at this point.

The rapid growth in the United States of university health sciences centers (academic health centers) is a positive force toward better collaboration among health professionals. The strong professionalism of each of the health professional groups cannot, however, be controlled only from within the university. It will have to be a national phenomenon and come from the consumers and their representatives.

V

PERSPECTIVES
ON EPIDEMIOLOGY
AND HEALTH STATISTICS
IN THE UNITED STATES

15

NEEDS AND OPPORTUNITIES
FOR ACTION

Problems and Issues: Discussion

Following presentation and discussion of the foregoing papers, the participants in the Conference on Epidemiology as a Fundamental Science in Health Services Planning, Administration, and Evaluation divided into four groups, each to consider the following series of questions:

1. What are the necessary conditions and settings for the preparation of contemporary epidemiologists and health statisticians in the short term and in the long term?

2. What are the necessary conditions and settings for employing the expertise of epidemiologists and health statisticians in the short term and in the long term?

3. What are the most effective means of promoting the education and training of epidemiologists and health statisticians in the short term and in the long term?

4. Who should be responsible for accomplishing these objectives?

5. What action should be taken now?

The results of the four group discussions were reported to the general session which concluded the conference. A summary of the substance of these reports follows.

Several issues were defined as central throughout all the discussion groups. The first is the problem of educating users or consumers of epidemiological knowledge or studies such as those in the political arena or government, as described by Dr. Anderson, and administrators of institutions or services at the community level. A second issue was how to achieve better cross-fertilization between epidemiology and other users of quantitative techniques in the analysis of health problems, that is, economics, sociology, and, in general, the management sciences. A third issue is the question of what should be added or what changes made in epidemiological training programs to improve their effectiveness and appeal. In this connection, a fourth issue is what can be done specifically to recruit more effectively for the field than has heretofore been the case. The fifth and most critical issue is the problem of the lack of teachers, both in numbers and in, perhaps, appropriate kinds of mixes of epidemiologists who can teach epidemiology as applied to health services planning and administration.

It was generally agreed that not only more of the same is needed, but that there is a need for a new breed of epidemiologist in the United States. The question at that point becomes, where can the new breed be developed? The settings, whether schools of public health, medical schools or elsewhere, must offer effective interfaces with the health care system, and in particular at the planning levels within the overall system. It was further specified that, to be effective, settings for the development of faculty must interact more effectively with all the health professional schools and with the university as a whole. These settings must serve as focal points where the total resources of the university can be made available, can be brought to bear on or in turn be available to the epidemiological scholar and to the generation of future epidemiological activities. In particular, there is clearly a great deal to be done to familiarize faculty and students of university health sciences centers with epidemiology and to establish conditions under which effective teaching and faculty development in this field can take place.

The basic concepts and methods used by the new breed of epidemiologist are identical to those of his colleagues, but the application of these techniques is quite different in that the new epidemiologists will function as one member of a team that will include administrators, planners, and other decision-makers. In preparation for this role the epidemiologist needs exposure to the broad range of "optimization" techniques as part of the educational process; it was suggested that a good portion of these optimization techniques are found in disciplines to which epidemiology is not traditionally related, for example, economics, management sciences, public administration, and political science.

Three kinds of epidemiological applications were outlined as a framework for further discussion. One is traditional, etiologically oriented epidemiology where the need to continue support for training and development is fully recognized. A second is epidemiology applied to health services research, development, and evaluation, also clearly in need of continued support. Most attention was paid to epidemiology in relation to decision-making with respect to resource allocation and the organization of health services. There was a strong sentiment to separate this use of epidemiology from traditional (academic) research epidemiology. In that context, specific note was made of the evident lack of political skills on the part of epidemiologists and of the need to provide these skills through education or by the selection process.

There was also discussion of the need to provide health training programs in other disciplines that would be working closely with epidemiologists. It was noted that the most critical training needs at the present time are for epidemiologists, medical economists, and medical sociologists. Although the statutory authority for training programs in these fields does, in fact, exist, no money has been appropriated. This constitutes a crippling problem; without trained manpower in these fields, little can be accomplished. There is a truly urgent need to prepare for the impact of the growing scarcity of health resources, mainly on decision-making throughout the health services system in the United States; epidemiology, more than most disciplines, has a great deal to contribute in illuminating that process. This obvious need adds to the sense of urgency in resolving the problems of developing effective strategies for improving teaching and practice in this discipline in the near future.

One of the areas to which epidemiology needs to turn its attention more effectively is its role in pointing out which efficacious resources designed to improve health should be promoted, that is, the identification of priorities. Once these have been pointed out, the final decisions will be made through the political process, based on the information supplied. In discussing short-term and long-term needs, major focus was placed on the short term, where there is much need for curriculum development and new recruitment techniques, to be supported on a large scale. This must of necessity be done before the effects of long-range training programs can be observed. The long run is also dependent upon stable financing mechanisms that are not presently available. Further, some evaluation mechanism to monitor the progress of training programs needs to be developed; these is none available at present.

Because the necessary faculty is not available and the curriculum content has not been fully specified, we cannot set out immediately to train the 2,000 or more of the new breed of epidemiologists needed now. Another short-term need clearly is to reach people who are concerned with decision-making at the community and operating levels, perhaps by a national approach similar to the one developed in Canada by Mc-Master University as the Health Care Evaluation Seminar. These and other short-term techniques need to be aggressively pursued. Finally, a task force needs to be created promptly to bring together epidemiologists, health planners, health researchers, people responsible for their employment, and potential funding sources to look for ways in which development of this field could be accelerated.

Concluding Comments

Summary of Comments by E. George Knox, M.D.

I would like to react to the issues raised in discussion by making four separate points.

    1. There is a pressing need to identify the administrative levels from which developments in epidemiology and health care studies are to be promoted and supported. Proper planning always requires realistic and accurate knowledge of where the point of decision lies and on assurance that powers of implementation exist; these do not seem to have been established during the course of this conference.

    2. I would like to develop a point raised by Professor McKeown concerning the two parallel developments which tend to occur in the evolution of health services; one is concerned with the way health services are financed and the other with the kinds of health services to be delivered. When one is deeply involved in one kind of development

there may be a tendency to inhibit movement in the other area; one kind of change at one time is enough for most people. This may provide a problem in the United States, as it did in Great Britain in 1948, in that the legislation currently being considered is concerned primarily with finance; this creates a danger that the health services themselves may fossilize in the mold of the moment. A great deal of planning and forethought needs to be given to the prevention of this fossilization process.

3. The question of the supply of and the demand for epidemiologists and training facilities has been raised repeatedly during this conference. There is nothing at all wrong with the tradition and quality of epidemiologists in the United States except that several speakers have suggested that there is an acute shortage and perhaps that there is a particular shortage of activity in the field of health care studies. I suggest that this is too simple a picture and that we need to add another dimension to the problem of supply and demand. Following reorganization of the National Health Service we have in Great Britain both a shortage and an excess in the sense that there are too many people looking for new jobs and not enough people with the necessary qualifications to fill the available jobs. That is, the pattern of duties has changed following the reorganization, and the retraining program has not yet caught up with the changed situation. Although the question of oversupply does not seem to be a problem in the United States at the moment, the establishment of a greater training service without the creation of appropriate jobs to occupy the trainees could result at the very least in an administrative problem and a form of oversupply. The response to this situation in Great Britain has been reasonably logical in that a series of job specifications were written for the various kinds of community health specialists outlining the locations and contents of their day-to-day occupations. We do not yet know how these specifications will work out in practice but there is certainly much justification for attempting to prepare them and for fitting the initial training program to their requirements.

4. Finally, I should like to offer some guidelines on the grammar of any recommendation. Three points are involved: first, a recommendation must define what is to be done; second, the verbs used for this definition must be verbs of visible action, preferably with visible outcomes, so that the successful completion of objectives can be ascertained; and third, a recommendation must designate who will perform the action. I hope that a recommendation formulated along these lines will result from the present conference.

Summary of Comments by Donald O. Anderson, M.D.

During this conference comments have come from all sides on the difficulty of defining epidemiology, a question that has been debated many times in the past. The problem is that there is an extremely small central core that is intrinsically epidemiological, probably comprising mainly the logic of science, which can be taught very quickly. I mentioned earlier the possibility that this core can be taught in six or seven hours. We have to do that in medical schools, because that is all the time the faculty is willing to allocate to teaching the scientific method. Each of us adds onto the core various other creations that we draw from other disciplines, such as microbiology, sociology, statistics, computer science, information science, systems analysis, the list goes on and on, meaning that each one of us as an epidemiologist is a different "flower child" of some sort or other. We are each our own peculiar breed; no two of us are exactly alike because each one has had a different mix of these other disciplines added onto our epidemiological core. This is basic, and this is why we wrestle in the various journals of epidemiology over the logic of research; but what constitutes that logic is a peculiar mixture, partly our training, partly our predisposition, and partly the environment in which we work.

Therefore, another term needs to be created for what we are doing. The British have done so, by using words such as social medicine and by now creating the Faculty of Community Medicine. We in Canada have also used that term, defining it by stating that epidemiology, biometry, sociology, and administration form the core of "community-based" methods. Every epidemiologist is involved in that general area, but each one has different strengths that he brings to this discipline. It follows then that, because we are operating at multiple levels of rationality and experience, we will no doubt argue forever about the boundaries of epidemiology.

My second point is taken from Dr. Noralou P. Roos of the University of Manitoba Faculty of Medicine, who describes the relationship between the researcher and the medical administrator as a discordance between the validity of findings and the speed of responsiveness with which the findings have to be produced for the decision-maker (1). Dr. Roos points out that the administrator and the politician generally want data that are produced very rapidly, and will accept data of questionable validity because decisions have to be made immediately. On the other hand, those of us who like to do well considered scientific research operate at a different level: we want to emphasize highly valid research that is reproducible, but the time scale over which we do it may be our entire career. Dr. Roos points out that the compromise, made necessary by the system of financing, lies somewhere in between. We compromise between the validity of a controlled clinical trial, on the one hand, and the need to get a decision out to the decision-makers on screening procedures immediately because they have to make decisions in the political arena, on the other hand. The epidemiologist, as health services planner, has many roles to play as a result of this. If he tends to concentrate on one level he is clearly an agent for change. If he is operating somewhere in the middle, he is clearly playing the role of an advocate for change. If he is operating at another level, he clearly is demonstrating the need for change. If he monitors change itself, another dimension, he is a monitor of change. If he keeps his data bases and merely observes what happens, he may be blind to change, spending his entire life involved in something that is purely esoteric and of little practical validity. In practice, each one of us keeps shifting our styles and roles, depending upon the development of our research careers, because we have different skills and different bags of tricks that we bring to the logic of science. This creates the need for an organization such as the International Epidemiological Association, in the United States the Association of Teachers of Preventive Medicine, or in Canada the Canadian Association of Teachers of Social and Preventive Medicine, in order to tie together the groups that are practicing social medicine. This brings me, then, to advocate the need for an epidemiological imagination, held by people who can shift in their perspective as they feel science is ready to shift; who are developing and exploiting the principles of social medicine.

A topic emphasized by a number of discussions has been the training programs. We can only teach epidemiology by demonstrating how to do it. There is no theory in what we have been discussing because the central core of epidemiology can be taught very easily, and our students must learn by observing how we apply epidemiology in reality at different levels of the social system. This means, then, training programs in which the university is intimately involved in playing a role in society. We all share with the students the projects that we are involved in, but if we are involved in pursuing by epidemiological principles something to the nth degree and remain blind to the need for change, our students will come away with different perceptions of the value of epidemiology than will students seeing how their professors are applying epidemiology to bring about social change. Epidemiologists must become involved in the planning process and share that planning experience with the students.

This brings us to something noted by Walter McNerney: perhaps the time has come for all of us to begin to change the system and to develop corporate planning structures. Planning has come about in Canada in the last few years for several reasons, among them a lack of money. It became necessary to talk about cost-benefit and cost-effectiveness, and the very use of those words demanded epidemiological input. It was also because of the federal leadership and its desire to change the planning structures so that the Federal Government could more easily free money to the provinces for specific purposes. Perhaps also planning is coming about because of our liberal reformist tradition, which shows itself in the election of new provincial governments which then provide opportunities for our students and professors to become involved in planning.

However, can this be captured and institutionalized without destroying it in a corporate planning system? Here is where we in Canada have to look for guidance in the United States. Clearly, we must put money into the agencies for planning, which indicates that the time has come to train epidemiologists and managers together. This is being done at the University of British Columbia where, with other colleagues, Dr. Anne Crichton, a sociologist, and I together teach health services planning. Dr. Crichton emphasizes management skills and the political structures of society and analyzes my actions. I teach her and the students the quantitative tools of planning. Together we are training a new breed of planners who, with a common training, half of which is in management and half in research, are graduating to take up positions in the Canadian planning infrastructures.

The last point that seems to have emerged from what has been said here is that the time has come for us to begin to put this sort of thing on paper, to develop a guide that will explain the role of epidemiology in health services planning and will provide a way of sharing our experiences and our curricula and of developing the conceptualization of this newly emerging kind of social medicine cum-epidemiology, cum-planning. Such is the function of organizations like the International Epidemiological Association, to pull us together and, through sharing, to help us to understand what we are all about.

Reference

1. N. P. Roos, "Evaluation, Quasi-Experimentation, and Public Policy," in *Quasi-Experimental Approaches,* ed. J. A. Caporaso and L. L. Roos, Jr. (Evanston, Ill.: Northwestern Univ. Press, 1973), pp. 281–304.

Concluding Statement

Frederick C. Robbins, M.D.

Recent developments in public health policy and federal legislation place new responsibilities on the health sciences professions. Schools of public health and universities with health sciences centers must relate themselves to the field of health services planning and the manpower needs identified at this conference much more directly than they have in the past. Changes are urgently needed in attitudes on the part of those who teach and practice clinical medicine with respect to the importance of epidemiological concepts and community health care problems. We believe that the Association of American Medical Colleges should take the lead in exploring ways and means to improve the teaching of epidemiology and community medicine in the medical schools of the United States. Specific priorities should be placed on recruiting and training persons who are not only psychologically prepared, but equipped with specific skills, to enter the fields of epidemiology, community medicine, and health services research.

Other professional organizations should assume similar leadership roles on behalf of their constituents. Follow-up efforts should be directed at defining job descriptions and careers more precisely and at identifying educational objectives and the kinds of training programs needed. Within the medical schools and health sciences centers of this country, the importance of these needs is beginning to filter through and in many schools there is considerable ferment, but the stimulus has come largely from the outside, from government, from citizens' groups, and from those who control the flow of funds. We have an opportunity that must be taken very seriously and developed vigorously.

Statement by the Conference

1. Until very recently in the United States there have been few constraints on health care resources, no effective planning processes that relate the flow of funds for manpower and capital to community needs, and no clear foci of responsibility and accountability. Therefore, there has been no obvious need and little incentive for the practical application of epidemiological skills and for the development of adequate health services management personnel and health information systems.

2. The recent federal PSRO legislation, the Health Services Research, Health Statistics and Medical Libraries Act, and the Health Planning and Resources Development Act have dramatically changed this situation. Each new PSRO, Health Systems Agency, and State Health Development Authority now being established will require personnel with epidemiological and management skills as well as clinical experience, and a mutual understanding of the interrelationships between these skills.

3. The discipline of epidemiology, together with the applied fields of economics, management sciences, and the social sciences, provide the essential quantitative and analytical methods, principles of logical inquiry, and rules for evidence for:

investigating the natural history of disease;

diagnosing, measuring, and projecting the health needs of communities and populations;

determining health goals, objectives, and priorities;

allocating and managing health care resources;

assessing intervention strategies and evaluating the impact of health services.

4. The United States does not currently have adequate epidemiological and management personnel and the necessary coordinated information systems to support these new federal legislative initiatives. Few medical schools, health sciences centers, or other university health programs are providing their graduates with a sufficient background in epidemiological methods, management science, and related disciplines to prepare them for roles of leadership in the new community agencies for the planning, administration, and evaluation of health services.

5. There is an urgent short-term as well as long-term need to train individuals in these areas. This will require the development of short-term courses to provide a basic level of competency for initial staffing of the planning agencies in addition to new and expanded educational programs to meet the long-term aspirations of the legislation. All appropriate educational settings should be involved in this effort.

6. The conference calls upon all interested professional organizations and public and private groups to discuss and further define the needs for new health services personnel identified at the meeting, and to work together in developing the necessary training programs and educational opportunities, by means of discussions, task forces, or follow-up conferences. In particular, the conference urges that a lead role be played by the Association of American Medical Colleges, the Coordinating Council on Medical Education, the American Medical Association, the American Association of Dental Schools, the Association of Schools of Public Health, the Association of University Programs in Health Adminis-

tration, the American Hospital Association, the Commission on Human Resources of the National Research Council, the Institute of Medicine, the Health Resources Administration of the Department of Health, Education and Welfare, the legislative staffs of the Congressional committees, and interested foundations.

Hunt Valley Inn
Baltimore, Maryland
March 4, 1975

APPENDICES

Participants in the Conference on Epidemiology as a Fundamental Science in Health Services Planning, Administration, and Evaluation

Contributors

Roy M. Acheson, M.D.

Donald O. Anderson, M.D.

Robert L. Berg, M.D.

John Cassel, M.D.

John Evans, M.D.

Susie Gilderdale

Alan Gittelsohn, Ph.D.

J. Thomas Grayston, M.D.

Maureen M. Henderson, M.D.

Basil S. Hetzel, M.D.

Walter W. Holland, M.D.

E. George Knox, M.D.

Jan Kostrzewski, M.D.

Adetokunbo O. Lucas, M.D.

Louis M. F. Massé, M.D.

Thomas McKeown, M.D.

Walter McNerney

Edward A. Mortimer, M.D.

Johannes Mosbech, M.D.

Herman A. Tyroler, M.D.

W. Estlin Waters, M.B.

Kerr L. White, M.D.

Session Chairmen

John C. Greene, D.D.S.

Margaret Mahoney

Edward B. Perrin, Ph.D.

Frederick C. Robbins, M.D.

Group Chairmen and Rapporteurs

Richard A. Berman

Roger J. Bulger, M.D.

Harry P. Cain, II, Ph.D.

Frederick V. Featherstone, M.D.

Gary L. Filerman, Ph.D.

Manfred Pflanz, M.D.

David J. Sencer, M.D.

August G. Swanson, M.D.

Invited Participants

Roy M. Acheson, M.D.
Director, Centre for Extension Training
in Community Medicine
London School of Hygiene and Tropical Medicine
31 Bedford Square
London WC1B, 3EL, England

Donald O. Anderson, M.D.
Health Sciences Centre
Director, Division of Health Services
Research and Development
IRC Building
The University of British Columbia
Vancouver, B.C. V6T JW5, Canada

Bertha D. Atelsek
Acting Director, Division of Health
Services Quality Research
National Center for Health Services
Research
Department of Health, Education, and
Welfare
5600 Fishers Lane
Rockville, Maryland   20852

Robert L. Berg, M.D.
Professor and Chairman
Department of Preventive Medicine
and Community Health
School of Medicine and Dentistry
The University of Rochester
260 Crittenden Boulevard
Rochester, New York   14642

Richard A. Berman
Assistant Dean and Associate Hospital
Director for Ambulatory Care
Services
The New York Hospital-Cornell Medical Center
525 East 68th Street
New York, New York   10021

Jan E. Blanpain, M.D.
Professor and Director
Department of Hospital Administration
and Medical Care Organization
School of Public Health
Vital Decosterstraat 102
3000 Leuven, Belgium

Roger Bulger, M.D.
Executive Officer
Institute of Medicine
National Academy of Sciences
2101 Constitution Avenue
Washington, D.C.   20418

Harry P. Cain, II, Ph.D.
Acting Director, Bureau of Health
Planning and Resources
Development
Health Resources Administration
Department of Health, Education and
Welfare
5600 Fishers Lane
Rockville, Maryland   20852

Richard Cash, M.D.
Instructor of Social and Preventive
Medicine
University of Maryland School of
Medicine
31 S. Greene Street
Baltimore, Maryland   21201

John Cassel, M.D.
Alumni Distinguished Professor
Department of Epidemiology
School of Public Health
University of North Carolina
Chapel Hill, North Carolina   27514

Nicholas Cavarocchi
Labor-HEW Subcommittee
Committee on Appropriations
House of Representatives
Rayburn Building
Washington, D.C.   20515

John A. D. Cooper, M.D.
President, Association of American Medical Colleges
One Dupont Circle, N.W.
Washington, D.C. 20036

Harley M. Dirks
Committee on Appropriations
United States Senate
Washington, D.C. 20510

Thomas Dublin, M.D.
Special Assistant to the Deputy Director
Bureau of Health Manpower
Department of Health, Education and Welfare
9000 Rockville Pike
Bethesda, Maryland 20014

Paul S. Ehrlich, Jr., M.D.
Director, Office of International Health
Office of the Assistant Secretary for Health
Parklawn Building
5600 Fishers Lane
Rockville, Maryland 20852

Kenneth M. Endicott, M.D.
Administrator, Health Resources Administration
Department of Health, Education and Welfare
5600 Fishers Lane
Rockville, Maryland 20852

John Evans, M.D.
President
The University of Toronto
Toronto, Canada M5S 1A1

Frederick V. Featherstone, M.D.
Program Director
W. K. Kellogg Foundation
400 North Avenue
Battle Creek, Michigan 49016

Jacob J. Feldman, Ph.D.
Acting Associate Director for Analysis
National Center for Health Statistics
Department of Health, Education and Welfare
5600 Fishers Lane
Rockville, Maryland 20852

Gary L. Filerman, Ph.D.
Executive Director
Association of University Programs in Health Administration
One Dupont Circle, N.W.
Washington, D.C. 20036

Gail Fisher
Acting Associate Director for the Cooperative Health Statistics System
National Center for Health Statistics
Department of Health, Education and Welfare
5600 Fishers Lane
Rockville, Maryland 20852

Reginald Fitz, M.D.
Senior Medical Associate
The Commonwealth Fund
Harkness House
1 East 75th Street
New York, New York 10021

Peter Fox
Director for the Office of Health Analysis
Office of the Assistant Secretary for Planning and Evaluation
Department of Health, Education and Welfare
330 Independence Avenue, S.W.
Washington, D.C. 20201

Donald J. Galagan, D.D.S.
Executive Director
American Association of Dental Schools
1625 Massachusetts Avenue, N.W.
Washington, D.C. 20036

Eli Ginzberg, Ph.D.
Director, Conservation of Human Re-
sources Project
Columbia University
New York, New York   10027

Alan Gittelsohn, Ph.D.
Professor of Biostatistics
School of Hygiene and Public Health
The Johns Hopkins University
615 N. Wolfe Street
Baltimore, Maryland   21205

Robert J. Glaser, M.D.
President, The Henry J. Kaiser Family
Foundation
2 Palo Alto Square
Palo Alto, California   94304

LeRoy Goldman
Committee on Labor and Public
Welfare
United States Senate
Washington, D.C.   20510

J. Thomas Grayston, M.D.
Vice President for Health Affairs
University of Washington Health Sci-
ences Center
Seattle, Washington   98195

John Greene, D.D.S.
Special Assistant for Dental Affairs
Office of the Assistant Secretary for
Health
Department of Health, Education and
Welfare
5600 Fishers Lane
Rockville, Maryland   20852

Scott Greer, Ph.D.
Senior Adviser for Social Science
Office of Scientific Affairs
Health Resources Administration
Department of Health, Education and
Welfare
5600 Fishers Lane
Rockville, Maryland   20852

Jean-Pierre Habicht, M.D.
Special Assistant to the Director
Division of Health Examination Sta-
tistics
National Center for Health Statistics
Department of Health, Education and
Welfare
5600 Fishers Lane
Rockville, Maryland   20852

Tom Hatch
Director, Division of Associated Health
Professions
Bureau of Health Manpower
Department of Health, Education and
Welfare
7550 Wisconsin Avenue
Bethesda, Maryland   20014

Maureen Henderson, M.D.
Professor and Chairman
Department of Social and Preventive
Medicine
University of Maryland School of
Medicine
Baltimore, Maryland   21201
Present address:
University of Washington Health Sci-
ences Center
Seattle, Washington   98195

Basil S. Hetzel, M.D.
Professor of Social and Preventive
Medicine
Monash University—Alfred Hospital
Melbourne, Australia 3181

Howard H. Hiatt, M.D.
Dean, Harvard School of Public Health
677 Huntington Avenue
Boston, Massachusetts   02115

Walter W. Holland, M.D.
Professor of Clinical Epidemiology and
Social Medicine
St. Thomas's Hospital Medical School
London, SE1, 7EH, England

Barbara Hulka, M.D.
Associate Professor of Epidemiology
School of Public Health
University of North Carolina
Chapel Hill, North Carolina   27514

David Kindig, M.D.
Deputy Director
Bureau of Health Manpower
Department of Health, Education and
    Welfare
9000 Rockville Pike
Bethesda, Maryland   20014

Ronald M. Klar, M.D.
Deputy Director
Bureau of Health Manpower
Department of Health, Education and
    Welfare
5600 Fishers Lane
Rockville, Maryland   20852

E. George Knox, M.D.
Director, Health Services Research
    Centre
University of Birmingham
Edgbaston, Birmingham B15 2TG,
    England

Robert Knouss, M.D.
Director, Division of Medicine
Bureau of Health Manpower
Department of Health, Education and
    Welfare
9000 Rockville Pike
Bethesda, Maryland   20014

Jan Kostrzewski, M.D.
Chief, Department of Epidemiology
State Institute of Hygiene
Chocimska 24
Warsaw 36, Poland

John T. Law
Executive Director
The Hospital for Sick Children
555 University Avenue
Toronto, Ont., Canada

Paul Leaverton, Ph.D.
Acting Associate Director for Statistical
    Research
National Center for Health Statistics
Department of Health, Education and
    Welfare
5600 Fishers Lane
Rockville, Maryland   20852

Charles E. Lewis, M.D.
Professor of Medicine and Public
    Health
School of Public Health
University of California
Los Angeles, California   90053

Betty A. Lockett, Ph.D.
Chief, International Study Staff
Division of Medicine
Bureau of Health Manpower
Department of Health, Education, and
    Welfare
9000 Rockville Pike
Bethesda, Maryland   20014

Adetokunbo O. Lucas, M.D.
Professor of Social and Preventive
    Medicine
University of Ibadan
Ibadan, Nigeria

William A. Lybrand, Ph.D.
Associate Administrator for Scientific
    Affairs
Office of Scientific Affairs
Health Resources Administration
Department of Health, Education and
    Welfare
5600 Fishers Lane
Rockville, Maryland   20852

Margaret Mahoney
Vice President
The Robert Wood Johnson Foundation
Princeton, New Jersey   08540

Harold Margulies, M.D.
Deputy Director
Health Resources Administration
Department of Health, Education and
    Welfare
5600 Fishers Lane
Rockville, Maryland   20852

Louis M. F. Massé, M.D.
Professeur à l'Ecole
Nationale de la Santé Publique
35043 Rennes, France

Thomas McCarthy, Ph.D.
Assistant Administrator for Systems
Liaison
Health Resources Administration
Department of Health, Education and
Welfare
5600 Fishers Lane
Rockville, Maryland 20852

Fred R. McCrumb, M.D. (deceased)
Special Assistant to the Director
Fogarty International Center
National Institutes of Health
Bethesda, Maryland 20014

Thomas McKeown, M.D.
Department of Social Medicine
University of Birmingham
Birmingham, England B15 2TJ

Gordon McLachlan
Secretary
Nuffield Provincial Hospitals Trust
3 Prince Albert Road
London N.W.1, 7SP, England

Walter McNerney
President, Blue Cross Association
840 North Lake Shore Drive
Chicago, Illinois 60611

Judith Miller
Health Staff Seminar
1901 Pennsylvania Avenue, N.W.
Washington, D.C. 20006

Edward Mortimer, M.D.
Professor and Chairman
Department of Community Medicine
Case Western Reserve University
2109 Adelbert Road
Cleveland, Ohio 44106

Johannes Mosbech, M. D.
Department of Medicine
Copenhagen County Hospital
2300 Copenhagen
Denmark

Jane H. Murnaghan
Assistant Professor of Health Care
Organization
School of Hygiene and Public Health
The Johns Hopkins University
615 N. Wolfe Street
Baltimore, Maryland 21205

Arthur D. Nelson, M.D.
President, American Board of Family
Practice
7301 East Fourth Street
Scottsdale, Arizona 85251

Andrew Pattullo
Vice President—Programs
W. K. Kellogg Foundation
400 North Avenue
Battle Creek, Michigan 49106

Mark Pearlman, M.D.
Division of Health Care Information
Systems and Technology
National Center for Health Services
Research
Department of Health, Education and
Welfare
5600 Fishers Lane
Rockville, Maryland 20852

Edward B. Perrin, Ph.D.
Professor, Department of Biostatistics
School of Medicine
University of Washington
Seattle, Washington 98195
(formerly Director, National Center for
Health Statistics)

Brad Perry, Ph.D.
Special Assistant to the Associate Di-
rector
Office of Academic and Intergovern-
mental Affairs
National Center for Health Services
Research
Department of Health, Education and
Welfare
5600 Fishers Lane
Rockville, Maryland 20852

Manfred Pflanz, M.D.
Visiting Professor
Department of Clinical Medicine and
  Health Care
University of Connecticut School of
  Medicine
Hartford Plaza
Hartford, Connecticut   06105

G. A. Phalp, CBE
Secretary, King Edward's Hospital Fund
  for London
14 Palace Court
London W2 4HT, England

Joseph de la Puente
Chief, Health Services Research Meth-
  ods Branch
Division of Health Services Research
  and Analysis
National Center for Health Services Re-
  search
Department of Health, Education and
  Welfare
5600 Fishers Lane
Rockville, Maryland   20852

Gerald Rosenthal, Ph.D.
Director, National Center for Health
  Services Research
Department of Health, Education and
  Welfare
5600 Fishers Lane
Rockville, Maryland   20852

Frederick C. Robbins, M.D.
Dean, School of Medicine
Case Western Reserve University
2119 Abington Road
Cleveland, Ohio   44106

Simone Sandier
CREDOC
Division d'Economie Médicale
45 Boulevard de la Gare
Paris XIII, France

Jessie M. Scott
Director, Division of Nursing
Bureau of Health Manpower
Department of Health, Education and
  Welfare
7550 Wisconsin Avenue
Bethesda, Maryland   20014

Isadore Seeman
Director, Division of Health Evaluation
Office of the Deputy Assistant Secre-
  tary for Health Planning and Analysis
Department of Health, Education, and
  Welfare
330 Independence Avenue, S.W.
Washington, D.C.   20201

David J. Sencer, M.D.
Director, Center for Disease Control
1600 Clifton Road, N.E.
Atlanta, Georgia   30333

James Shanks
President
The Rosslyn Foundation
1901 N. Fort Myer Drive
Rosslyn, Virginia   22209

Henry E. Simmons, M.D.
Office of the Assistant Secretary for
  Health
Department of Health, Education, and
  Welfare
330 Independence Avenue, S.W.
Washington, D.C.   20201

Eleanor Smith, M.D.
Health Care Financing Branch
Division of Health Systems Design and
  Development
National Center for Health Services
  Research
Department of Health, Education and
  Welfare
5600 Fishers Lane
Rockville, Maryland   20852

August G. Swanson, M.D.
Director of Academic Affairs
Association of American Medical
    Colleges
One Dupont Circle, N.W.
Washington, D.C.   20036

H. A. Tyroler, M.D.
Professor of Epidemiology
School of Public Health
University of North Carolina
Chapel Hill, North Carolina   27514

Robert van Hoek, M.D.
Acting Administrator
Health Services Administration
Department of Health, Education and
    Welfare
5600 Fishers Lane
Rockville, Maryland   20852

Homer Wadsworth
The Cleveland Foundation
Greater Cleveland Associated Foun-
    dation
700 National City Bank Building
Cleveland, Ohio   44114

Stanley S. Wallack
Director of the Office of Health Re-
    sources
Office of the Assistant Secretary for
    Planning and Evaluation
Department of Health, Education and
    Welfare
330 Independence Avenue, S.W.
Washington, D.C.   20201

W. Estlin Waters, M.B.
Professor and Head
Department of Community Medicine
Faculty of Medicine
Southampton General Hospital
Southampton S09 4XY, England

M. Keith Weikel, Ph.D.
Commissioner, Medical Services Ad-
    ministration
Social and Rehabilitation Service
Department of Health, Education and
    Welfare
330 C Street, S.W.
Washington, D.C.   20201

Kerr L. White, M.D.
Professor of Health Care Organization
School of Hygiene and Public Health
The Johns Hopkins University
615 N. Wolfe Street
Baltimore, Maryland   21205

Daniel F. Whiteside, D.D.S.
Director, Bureau of Health Manpower
Department of Health, Education and
    Welfare
9000 Rockville Pike
Bethesda, Maryland   20014

Claus A. Wirsig
Executive Director
University Teaching Hospitals Associa-
    tion
1300 Yonge Street
Toronto, Ont., M4T 1X3, Canada

Karl Yordy
Senior Program Officer
Institute of Medicine
National Academy of Sciences
2101 Constitution Avenue
Washington, D.C.   20418

Daniel I. Zwick
Associate Administrator for Planning,
    Evaluation, and Legislation
Health Resources Administration
Department of Health, Education and
    Welfare
5600 Fishers Lane
Rockville, Maryland   20852

INDEX